S0-BWL-996

Walking Wisdom
For Women

Walking Wisdom *For* Women

Plus+ing Your Walk
For Fitness, Career & Romance

by
Elaine P. Ward

Illustrations by
Bob Young

N.A.R.F. Publishing, Pasadena, CA

Walking Wisdom For Women
Plus+ing Your Walk
For Fitness, Career and Romance

Published by:
    N.A.R.F. Publishing
    Post Office Box 50312
    Pasadena, CA 91115-0312
    Tel/Fax: 818-577-2264

All rights reserved. No part of this book may be reproduced or transmitted in any form or by any means, electronic or mechanical, including photo-copying, recording or by any information storage and retrieval system with-out written permission from the author, except for the inclusion of brief quo-tations in a review.

Copyright ©1996, Elaine P. Ward
First Printing 1996
LC

Publisher's Cataloging in Publication
  (Prepared by Quality Books, Inc.)
Ward, Elaine P.
    Walking wisdom for women : plus+ing your walk for fitness, career & romance / Elaine P. Ward -- 1st ed.
      p.cm.
      Preassigned LCCN: 95-69495
      ISBN: 1-884647-02-2

      1. Walking (Sport) 1. Title
      GV1071.W37 1995
                       796.42'9
                       QBI95-20306

DEDICATION

*T*o my mother, Helen Hops, who at 89 regularly walks two to three miles a day. To my daughters, Daphne Gill and Laura McConnaughey, who as young mothers and working women, continue the family tradition of enthusiastic walkers.

ACKNOWLEDGEMENTS

*M*any people have been generous with their time and assistance in the preparation of this book. Most specifically, I would like to thank Bill Banks, Bud Herzberg and Casey Meyers for nudging me to make the transition between playing with the idea of the book and getting down to the serious effort of writing it. Lifelong appreciation to my brother, Ronald Pottenger, for always "being there" to lend mental and emotional support.

Thanks to Dori Devereux, Linda Meadow, Helen Powers, and Nancy Alexander for critiquing the manuscript at various levels of evolution. More thanks to Robert T. Pottenger, Jr., MD, Hugh Pendleton RTP, and Fred Smith for their professional comments and guidance. And, special thanks to Luanne Cad and Dee Anderson for photography.

Bouquets of roses go to Southern Cal Walkers -- Dee Anderson, Grace Burnham, Shirley Capps, Donna Cunningham, Carol Ferris, Marjorie Hanft, Helen Hops, Sat-Naryan Kaur, Barbara Kowalski, Shirley Lang, Ria Marsh, Linda Meadow, Carolyn Ryan, Virginia Scales, Mary Shudy, Joan Schlimgen, Sandra Williams, and Pat Willis.

Special recognition: Joanne Stevens Art & Design, South Pasadena, California.

ABOUT THE AUTHOR

*W*hen Elaine Ward was in her early forties, she discovered that she had a congenital lower back problem that interfered with her walking. After working with doctors and physical therapists, she met Frank Alongi, an internationally recognized racewalking coach. Frank taught her the biomechanics of efficient, safe walking, and she found that her own walking improved dramatically.

Wanting to share what she had learned with others, Elaine became a certified fitness and competitive walking instructor. She started giving walking classes and clinics for community colleges, hospitals and senior citizen's groups, and founded the Southern Cal Walkers, a fitness and competitive walking club for men and women.

Elaine is president of Walk Plus+ers and the managing director of Walk-Wise Walkers, a membership association for women. *WALKING WISDOM FOR WOMEN, Plus+ing Your Walk for Fitness, Career & Romance* is the product of 14 years of coaching women of all ages. She has received several national awards for her contributions as a walk leader.

Elaine also holds leadership positions in the Racewalking Committee of USA Track & Field and is the Managing Director of the North American Racewalking Foundation. She is the author of three books and a video on fitness and competitive walking, edits two national newsletters and writes a column for *Masters National News*, a track and field publication for athletes over 40.

Living in Southern California, Elaine is the grandmother of four boys and one girl. She thinks of her walking students as extended family and wants you to feel welcome to write to her at any time. Walk Plus+ers, 1000 San Pasqual, #35, Pasadena, CA 91106-3393.

ABOUT THE ILLUSTRATOR

*T*he drawings which enliven this book are by Bob Young. At age 55, Bob entered the rigorous illustration program at the Art Center College of Design in Pasadena, California, graduating with honors in 1992. His illustrations have appeared in the *New York Times, Modern Maturity, Harvard Magazine* and numerous other publications. He and his wife Sally, a librarian and teacher, share their home near Pasadena with two grand Bouvier dogs.

TABLE OF CONTENTS

—— FROM YOUR COACH ——

*Y*ou, yes YOU, can have a Great Walk... a walk that makes you feel good about yourself and makes others take notice....a walk that opens your life to new career opportunities and social fulfillment. It's there for you. All you have to do is "Go for it!"

Like most women, you probably recognize the importance of good health, a satisfying job, sex appeal and love. These values are at the top of most wish lists. They are the golden means that help you pursue and find happiness.

Here are some ways plus+ing your walk brings you more and better fitness, career success and romance.

++ PLUS+ING FOR FITNESS

+ You learn how to walk off extra pounds and look good doing it.

+ You are given tips for improving weak ankles, problem knees, aching shoulders and lower back pain.

+ You discover how to soothe inner stress by putting rhythm and comfort into your gait.

+ You are shown the essentials for making your fitness walking truly safe for your body.

+ You find out why putting technique into your walking takes some of the "work" out of workouts.

++ PLUS+ING FOR CAREER SUCCESS

+ You learn how to walk into a room and make a positive impression at job interviews and business meetings, even when you are anxious.

+ You discover that your walk can instill confidence in your boss, clients and customers.

+ You find that your walk can give you a competitive edge in getting a job promotion.

++ PLUS+ING FOR ROMANCE

+ You learn why some of the sexiest women have average bodies.

+ You are given tips for leveling the age barrier so you can have a youthful walk into your eighties.

+ You are shown ways of walking that attract attention to you, the person inside.

Plus+ing your walk definitely has a BIG plus sign. Plus+ing means adding to (even multiplying) the benefits in walking. You are introduced to many plus+ing factors — technique tips that make your walk a true and reliable asset, whether you are a regular fitness walker or an around-the-job-and-house walker.

THE PLAN

I

Helping you develop a Great Walk is the purpose of the plus+ing process. Section One humorously orients you to the two basic scientific principles affecting human walking. You have probably given little thought to how you walk, or how you look when you walk. It's a skill that goes on autopilot very early in life. Yet, walking habits tell tales, and it is wise to know their language.

II

In Section Two, you are guided to "see" yourself walking. You are introduced to the key elements of different types of posture, footwork, knee action, hip movement and arm swing to help you create your own walking portrait. By becoming aware of how you use your body, you are able to make the changes that give your walk a 10+ rating.

III

You are given the 12 technique tips of a Great Walk in Section Three. These tips take you through a walking makeover. Always keep in mind, an unattractive walk makes a negative statement that can frustrate your success in life. An attractive walk, on the other hand, can be one of your most helpful resources.

IV

In the Fourth Section, you are introduced to carefully selected limbering and strengthening exercises called plus+ers. Although proper walking technique feels good and looks good, a Great Walk has something more. It has the special vitality that springs from a fit body.

V

The final section reviews the payoffs you get from plus+ing your walk. With flourish and fanfare, you are then welcomed into the emerging elite of Great Walkers.

GO FOR IT!

Let me confess up front. I am a missionary about walking. I love to walk, and I want to add more fun and purpose to your walking. I want you to appreciate *all* a Great Walk can do for you. In your house, on the job, at the mall, in the park, along the roads and streets, you can plus your fitness, career and romantic life by practicing and playing with my technique tips. Fun is the operative word as you become involved in the plus+ing process. Enjoy, improve and prosper.

ORIENTATION

This just in!

Scientific sources report two extraordinary findings that are on the cutting edge of walking technology.

1. Human beings walk on two legs in an upright position.
2. Human beings are governed by the law of gravity.

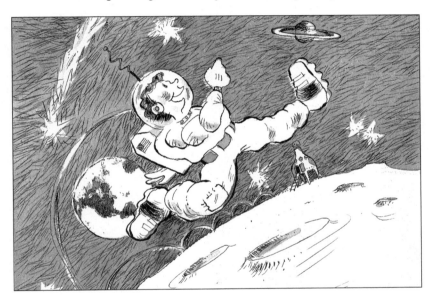

Ridiculous? Not at all! These findings mean that the fundamentals of correct walking are the same for everyone – at all ages, all sizes, shapes and speeds.

You started walking long before you can remember. You never doubted that you could walk. You simply began experimenting. At first, you settled for standing and balancing on your two feet. Then came the problem of coordinating your various body parts to move forward. Though there were "woops", "wobbles" and "thuds", it felt right to walk, and you gladly gave up crawling.

Because you never received any schooling about walking, you developed many subconscious habits as you grew up. Some of these habits were aided by genetic input. Some may have come from cultural influences and some were acquired by imitating others. The most revealing ones evolved from your feelings and thoughts about yourself.

Because walking became automatic early in life, you probably haven't thought much about how you walk now. You can't see yourself walking. You may hardly feel yourself walking. Can you answer these questions easily?

When you are walking:

How do you move your arms?

How do you hold your head?

How is your posture?

What direction are your toes pointed?

The ways you use the different parts of your body as you walk can be "for" or "against" you. They may be safe or stressful for your body. They may communicate positive or negative messages to others.

Just as it is smart to learn to use words accurately, it is smart to use correct technique when you walk. Well chosen words allow you to present yourself positively and to say what you mean. A well chosen walk allows you to present yourself confidently and influence others favorably.

You CAN take charge of your walk and maximize the fitness benefits you want. You CAN walk to your best advantage and communicate the right kind of messages to others.

WALKING WISDOM: Your walking habits tell tales. It is useful to know their language.

Now, try answering these questions:

When I am walking...

> Do I appear confident?
>
> Do I have sex appeal?
>
> Does my walk say "yes" to life, love and success?
>
> Am I a Julia Roberts or a Wilma Flintstone? A
> Katharine Hepburn or a Ma Kettle?*

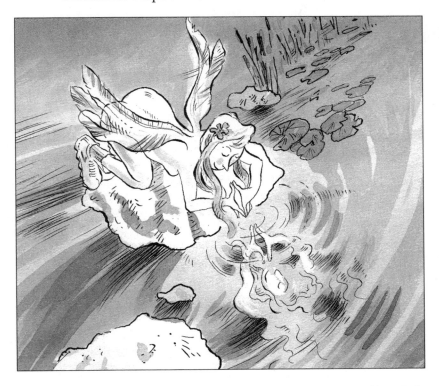

You get the picture. No one wants a blah walk. Blah scores 0. This is just as true for the 70-year-old as for the 20-year-old. Career success and romance are ageless. So is a Great Walk.

WALKING WISDOM: Be a turn-on, not a turn-off.

A Great Walk has proper biomechanics. It takes into consideration that we walk upright on two feet and are governed by the law of gravity. When you walk as nature intended, all of your body parts move efficiently with a minimum of wasted energy. As a consequence, a Great Walk feels good and looks smooth.

For those walking for fitness, the plus+ing technique synchronizes body movements and minimizes physical stress. For example, it reduces the stress on the lower back caused by uncoordinated arm and leg movements. It also reduces stress on the legs and knees caused by the feet slapping the ground at faster speeds.

For those seeking to climb the career ladder and earn more money, the plus+ing technique gives direction and purpose to body language. A Great Walk conveys the message, "I am someone worth betting on. I know where I am going and have the ability to get there."

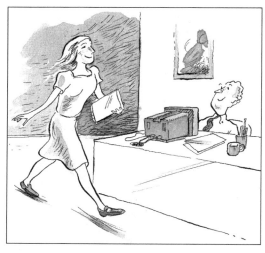

For those seeking romance, the plus+ing tips enhance sex appeal. They create a walk with a natural rhythm and style that is pleasing to watch. They also generate a dynamic of vitality that projects positive personality vibes to others and arouses interest in "getting to know you."

•● ●● **WALKING WISDOM: Many women identify with their children, job titles, cars and bank accounts. A smart woman also identifies with her walk.**

YOUR WALK
"As Is"

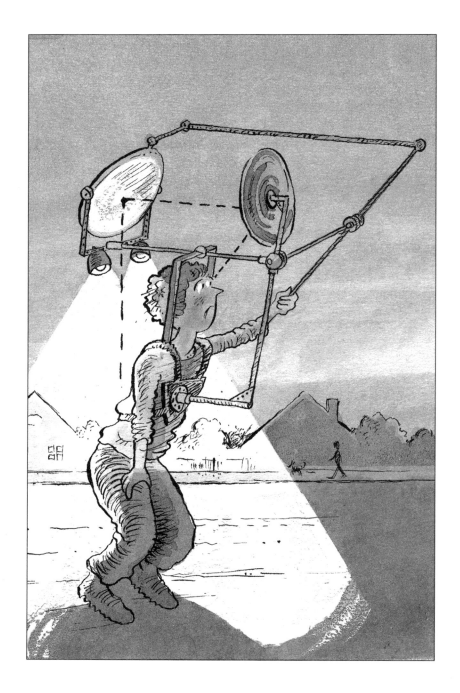

YOUR WALKING PORTRAIT

*Y*our first step along the plus+ing path is getting to know all about the way your body moves — from the soles of your feet to the crown of your head. This process of self-discovery is like looking in a mirror. You aren't always satisfied with what you see, but you know you can fix up.

In the following pages, you are given choices to help you describe the way you walk right now. You will use these choices to make a complete walking portrait. You may find it helpful to enlist a friend's eye or a video camera. When the given choices don't apply to you, write in your own descriptions.

You are also asked to note any orthopedic or other problems you may have that affect your walking. In fitness walking classes, extra weight, weak ankles, low back pain, and arthritis are common. After creating your walking portrait, you are given examples of how the plus+ing technique has helped some women manage their particular problems.

Fun and laughs await you as you start getting to know your walk. Let's begin at ground level with your feet.

THE FOOT
—Beast of Burden or Honored Friend

Praise the foot! Sturdy underpinning. Noble ground gripper. Exalted platform. Down-to-earth friend. Slider. Glider. Hopper. Skipper. Jumper. Stand-patter. Runner. And WALKER. Our closest point of contact with planet Earth.

Now, consider the uniqueness of your foot. Your foot is a highly specialized part of your body and has a distinctive design suited to walking upright. Contemplate your wondrous arch with its springy and resilient properties. No other walking, crawling, or flying species has a foot with an arch!

And don't forget: It was the foot of Neil Armstrong that took the "first giant step for mankind" on the surface of the moon. Your feet are hard to hug, but throw kisses at them for lugging you around. Then, observe how you use them as you walk.

❑ Both feet are straight.
❑ One foot toes out.
❑ Both feet toe out.
❑ One foot toes in.
❑ Both feet toe in.

My heel contacts the ground...

❑ in front of my body.
❑ close to my body.

Personal foot problem? _____

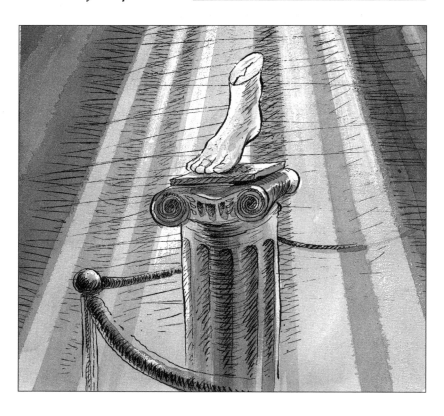

THE ANKLE

Your ankle may seem "down there", out-of-sight, but don't be fooled. It plays an important role in keeping you from falling on your face when you walk. By flexing your ankle toward your shin, your toes rise into the air and gain superiority over the uneven cracks and pits along the way.

How much you raise your toes affects the way you use your foot. If you barely flex your ankle, your foot comes down nearly flat. If you flex it more, your foot can roll smoothly from heel to toe.

Because of the ankle's function in walking, you need to know how strong and limber your ankles are.

My ankles are...
- ❑ strong and stable.
- ❑ weak and roll in (pronate).
- ❑ weak and roll out (supinate).
- ❑ limber.
- ❑ stiff.

Personal ankle problem? _____

THE KNEE
—Ignoble or Sublime

Your knee is a utilitarian hinge with an ingenious design for bending and withstanding stress. No poet has written a eulogy to the knee – though its uses are extraordinary!

Villains creep and grovel on their knees. The heavenly power of prayer and the ardent marriage proposal are intensified by kneeling. The knee is quite literally pivotal to many of our most dramatic activities.

Though the knee may be homely, even knobby, it significantly affects the style of a walk. A drum major straightens his legs to add dignity to his gliding gait. A hiker working against gravity uses the springing action of bent knees for upward thrust. Many fitness walkers have bounding, bent-knee strides.

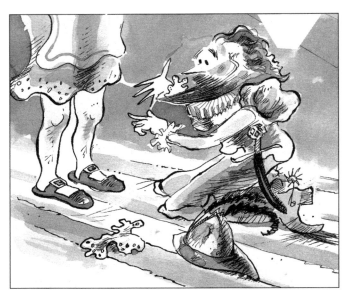

How shalt I compare thee, O KNEE?

How about YOUR knees?

To answer this question, walk a few steps and stop. Notice how one of your legs immediately comes under your body to bear your weight. It is in the support or vertical position.

Now, while you are walking, observe how your knee looks when your leg passes through the support position. (You may find this a good time to ask for someone's help.)

My knees are...

❑ very bent in the support position.
❑ somewhat bent in the support position.
❑ straight in the support position.

Personal knee problem? _____

THE TRUNK
—The Body's Suitcase

The trunk of your body is a sturdy suitcase. It holds and protects most of your vital organs. It also encases the spine - your body's central axis.

Many walkers look like their heads are stuck on trunks packed with cement. The only parts of their bodies that move are the arms and legs, and often the arms barely swing. Their clothing hangs motionless from their shoulders.

A rigid trunk is a sign that a walker has repressed his or her natural pelvic-hip rotation. Rather than rotating with the forward and backward movement of the legs, the pelvis and hips remain in place. Consequently, interaction between the movements of the upper body and lower body is inhibited.

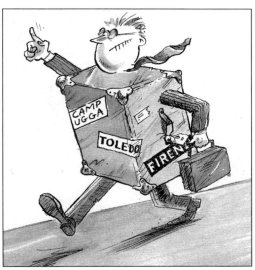

🚶 *Getting to know your pelvic-hip rotation:*

To see what is meant by pelvic hip rotation, stand in front of a mirror and put your hands around your waist. Rest your thumbs and index fingers on the bony edge of your pelvis. Turn your pelvis forward and backward and feel it moving under your fingers.

As you rotate your pelvis, look down toward your upper thighs. You will see that your hips are also turning back and forth. Because the pelvis and hips rotate together, when "hip rotation" is discussed, it will *always* mean pelvic-hip rotation in the plus+ing process. 🚶

Now ask yourself if your hips rotate as you walk? If you do not know, here is one way of finding out. Put on a pair of shorts or pants with a very visible, vertical seam on the outside. (You can use a piece of tape to substitute for a seam.) The span from just below your waist to the top of your leg is the area to watch. If you can see your seam moving back and forth as you walk, your hips are rotating. If there is no movement, they are not. (Again, a friend may be helpful here.)

Perhaps you feel action in your hips, but the seam of your shorts or pants does not shift. In this case, you may have a side-to-side tush swing rather than a back and forth hip rotation.

When I walk, my hips....
    ❑ do not rotate.
    ❑ rotate a little.
    ❑ swing side to side.
    ❑ turn back and forth freely.

Personal hip problem? _____

How does your back look and feel as you walk?
    ❑ slumped. (I feel tired all the time.)
    ❑ swayed.
    ❑ bent forward at the waist.
    ❑ bent backward at the waist.
    ❑ straight and stiff.
    ❑ straight and limber.

*Personal back problem?*_____

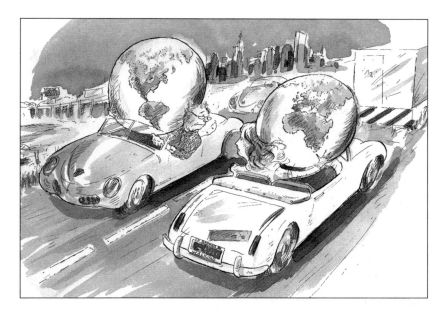

THE SHOULDER
—Atlas Syndrome. Ouch! My aching shoulders!

Like Atlas in Greek mythology, you may feel as though you have the weight of the world on your shoulders. Daily stresses and worldly cares accumulate and settle in your neck and shoulder muscles so they feel sore, tight and hard.

If you are a superwoman with a job and family, you are susceptible to the Atlas Syndrome. If you spend hours at a computer or drive in rush hour traffic, you are, too. As tight, achy shoulders affect movement, ask yourself: How do my shoulders feel when I am walking?

My shoulders are...
- ❏ pulled back and tense.
- ❏ slouched.
- ❏ raised and hard.
- ❏ sore and tight.
- ❏ relaxed.

*Personal shoulder problem?*_____

THE ARM

If you are anxious or self-doubting, you may hold your arms close to your sides and barely swing them as you walk. If you are happy, you may swing your arms freely. Many walkers swing both arms across their bodies as though massaging their stomachs, or they swing one arm across and the other forward.

Some Hindu gods have multiple arms. Imagine taking a walk with such an assembly. You are lucky to have only two.

How do my arms swing as I walk?
❑ across my body.
❑ one arm across, the other back and forth.
❑ my arms barely swing.
❑ back and forth at my sides.

*Personal arm problem?*_____

THE EXPRESSIVE HAND

Why do filmmakers so often zoom in on the hands? Probably they have many motives. The hands can express skill, dexterity, mastery and grace. They can appear clumsy and inept, or reveal arthritis and pain. Very importantly, they richly communicate human emotions in every day activities. Consider your hands when you are walking.

When I walk, my hands...
❑ are clenched.
❑ are stretched out
❑ hang limply.
❑ fidget.
❑ are relaxed.

Personal hand problem? _____

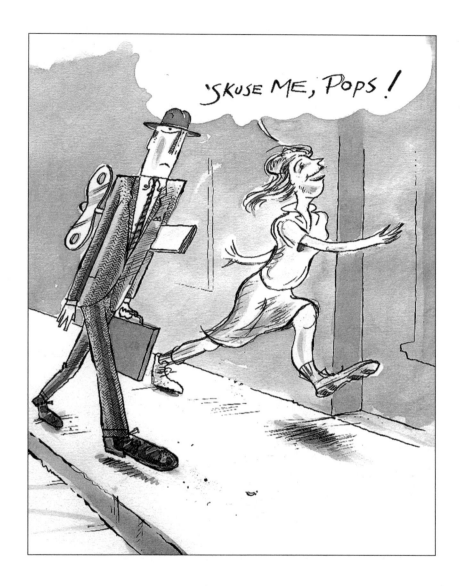

THE HEAD
—Crowning Glory

Your head with its big brain is your personal computer. It is your action center. It connects your senses to your thoughts, and your thoughts to your feelings. The way you carry your head and look out at the world is like an opening sentence. It gives an immediate impression of how you feel about yourself.

When you are walking, are you reasonably confident that the ground will stay put? Or do you feel you have to watch it to be sure? In other words, how do you usually hold your head?

I hold my head...
- ❏ up, eyes forward.
- ❏ bent back slightly.
- ❏ bent down with eyes on the ground.
- ❏ tilted to one side.
- ❏ thrust forward.

Personal head problem? _____

POSTURE
—Your Essential Theme

When you walk, you carry your body in a certain way. This way is your posture. The Victorians had a word for it: "Carriage." Posture gives your appearance design and style.

Casey Meyers in his definitive book, WALKING, A Complete Guide to The Complete Exercise, says, "Proper posture is absolutely, positively, unequivocally, without a doubt, the most critical, fundamental aspect of the walk." 1*

In spite of the importance of your posture, you may find the subject a bit boring. You may be a victim of the drill sergeant's approach to teaching children to "Stand up straight!"

1* Casey Meyers, WALKING, A Complete Guide to the Complete Exercise, (New York: Random House, 1992), p 80.

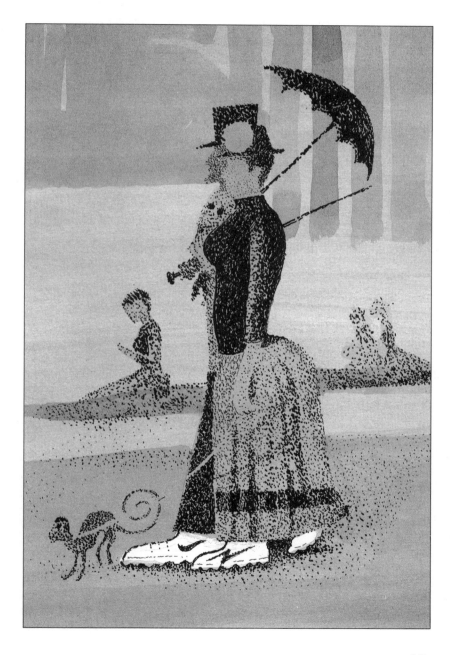

For a moment, consider your posture anew. Your posture affects your life continuously. It supports or undermines your fitness on a day-to-day basis. Also, it enhances or detracts from your appearance. Because your posture represents you constantly, you have every reason to wonder how good a job it does.

The following are five posture portraits. Check the one that is most like yours.

PERRRFECT POSTURE

For generations, erect, military posture was considered the ideal — head up, shoulders pulled back, chest thrust out, gut sucked in and buttocks tucked in. Demerits were given for any movement in the hips.

A woman was said to have good posture if she could balance a glass of water on her head without spilling a drop.

❑   My posture is Perrrfect.

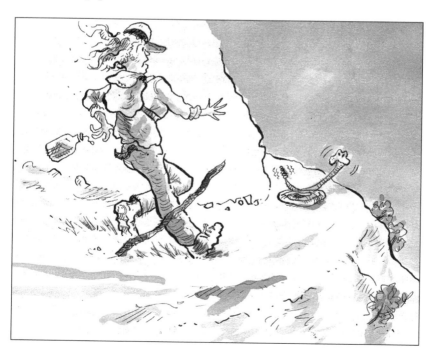

BACKWARD LEANER

Many walkers look like they are tipping backward. They stand with their weight on their heels, and they walk carrying invisible shoulder packs. Because of their reverse lean, gravity acts as a drag on their forward progress.

A backward lean makes sense for a timid hiker going down a Grand Canyon trail or for someone who has just surprised a snake, but ...

❑ I have an habitual backward lean.

SLOUCHER

Everyone—EVERYONE—knows what it is to slouch when tired or depressed, and that's okay. But how about all the time? The constant, caved-in, slouch walk appears to be halfway between a walk and a sit, or walk-sit. A sloucher makes a low, shambling statement, and gets a minus 10 rating on charisma.

❑ I walk with a slouch but have an excuse.

SWAYBACK

A swaybacked walk can feel sexy. For the guy, a swayback thrusts his chest and rear out, giving a rooster-like macho swagger. For the gal, it advertises the bust line and hips. One catch: A swayback is out-of-whack and can lead to chronic low back pain.

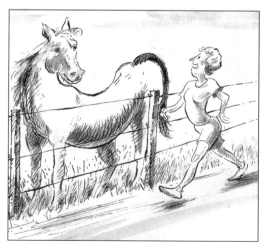

❑ That describes me.

FORWARD LEANER

The posture of a forward leaner is straight. The chest is lifted, and shoulders and neck are relaxed. When forward leaners walk, they use gravity to help them along. How? They maintain a slight lean from their ankles in the direction they are going.

❑ Forward leaners please Mother Nature.

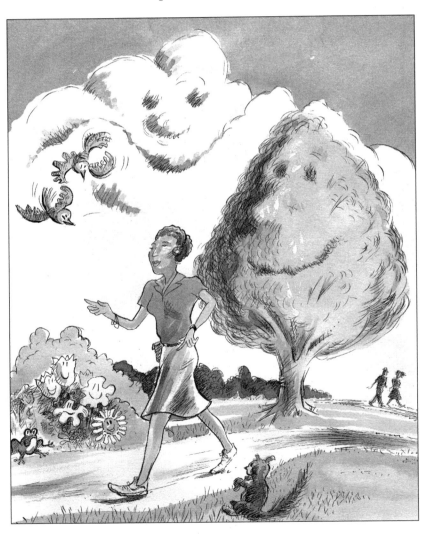

YOUR WALK *"As Is"*

Now that you have considered your posture and the use of the different parts of your body as you walk, it is time to assemble your complete walking portrait.

Think of yourself as a writer creating a verbal picture of yourself walking. You want to have the picture as true to life as possible to help you decide what elements in your walk need plus+ing. Look back at the choices you made in the previous pages, and transfer them to the appropriate lines below.

Feet_____

Ankles_____

Knees _____

Hips _____

Trunk_____

Shoulders_____

Arms_____

Head_____

Posture_____

Problems_____

_____

PLUS+ING COMMON PROBLEMS

Women often ask how the plus+ing technique helps manage weight and orthopedic problems. Here are eight true stories.

OVERWEIGHT: Peggy, a 32-year-old, was 60 pounds overweight when she came to class. She was strongly committed to losing weight and was on a doctor's program of exercise and diet. Initially, I gave her technique tips to exercise her waistline and arms. When she was comfortable with these tips, I showed her how to use her feet to give her legs and thighs more exercise. After twelve months, she had almost reached her weight goal. Her figure was firm and shaped, and her muscles were strong.

POOR CIRCULATION IN THE FEET: Mary, a 59-year-old, came to class and told me that her doctor was considering foot surgery. First, I told her to follow her doctor's final decision. Then, I showed her how to stimulate the circulation in her feet by plus+ing the way she used them. During the first class, she barely walked one-eighth of a mile. At the end of five weeks, she was able to walk a mile slowly and comfortably.

PROBLEM ANKLES AND KNEES: Two or three students in each walking class have weak and painful ankles or knees. By giving them plus+ing tips for strengthening these areas, many showed improvement just doing their daily, roundabout walking. Naturally, those who used the tips during regular fitness walks improved more quickly.

KNOCK-KNEES: A 10-year-old girl, Kerry, came to class with severely turned-in knees and ankles. Besides recommending proper shoes, I started her on some specific corrective exercises. (See Section Four.) After using these exercises, proper shoes, and the plus+ing footwork over a period of two years, Kerry was able to walk more normally.

ARTHRITIC HIPS: Helen, a 78-year-old widow, had arthritis in her left hip which came and went. When it came, she slowed her walking pace and modified the movement in her hips for a few days. In spite of these flare-ups, she was convinced that using the plus+ing technique with its gentle, limbering movements helped her stiffness and pain.

HIP REPLACEMENT: Paul, a 60-year-old dentist, came to class after having his right hip replaced. He had competed as a runner and swimmer in his younger years and wanted to try competitive walking. Because the plus+ing technique is good for all speeds, he kept to his goal and began entering races. He reported that he had no problem with his artificial hip.

LOWER BACK PAIN: Ginny, a mother and computer analyst, had mild to moderate low back pain from increasing scoliosis. With her doctor's encouragement, she began strengthening exercises for her abdominal muscles and gentle stretches for her lower back muscles. (See Plus+ers Section IV) At the same time, she corrected her walking posture and stressful arm movements. When she stopped class, she felt her back pain was better and was pursuing a goal of walking a 14 minute mile.

PAINFUL SHOULDERS: Nancy, a 48-year-old writer, complained of extremely tight and sore shoulder muscles. She blamed the long hours she spent at her computer. An all-or-nothing person, she became very serious about plus+ing her walk. After six weeks, she realized that her shoulder pain had lessened substantially. She credited her new arm swing for her recovery. She felt it massaged her shoulders every time she went fitness walking.

Now that you have learned how the plus+ing technique has helped some common problems, carefully consider any ones you may have. As you advance to the next part of your walking makeover, be sure the 12 plus+ing technique tips are safe for you. Check with your doctor. There is every reason to consider them safe; nonetheless, you are unique, and it's best to be certain.

If you cannot do some of the suggested tips, okay. Many fine walkers have limitations. By focusing on what you can do, you can develop the best walk possible for you — your own special Great Walk.

WALKING WISDOM: There is no perfection. There is always better.

PEOPLE WATCHING

Go to a busy street corner, and spend ten minutes just watching people walk. Notice their postures. Then, concentrate on how they use their feet, legs, hips and arms as well as on how they hold their heads. What kind of overall impressions do they make?

It won't take long before you start identifying different walking habits. You may get strong feelings about those you like and those you dislike.

WALKING WISDOM: A Great Walk and great jazz have something in common. They both depend on the blending of different parts.

PLUS+ING YOUR WALK

Into
A Great Walk

❧

THE PLUS+ING PROCESS

Each one of us is dealt certain cards that we must play throughout our lives. The fun and challenge in life is learning to play them well.

We may not have been dealt the body size or shape that we would like, but we can make the most of what we have. We may not possess the health we would like, but we can become surprisingly fit. Some things cannot be changed, but almost everything can be improved.

By plus+ing your walk into a Great Walk, you take control of a very visible part of your appearance. You turn one of your most available skills into a dependable asset that can serve you well.

•• •• WALKING WISDOM: The secret to a Great Walk is to catch the moonbeam called desire and reach for the star inside of you.

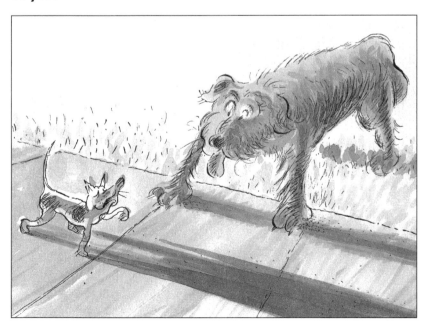

THE PLUS+ING TECHNIQUE

Playing golf requires technique. The same is true for bowling, tennis, skiing, horseback riding, gymnastics, swimming .... and walking. Like any skill, walking can be done well or so-so.

Would you settle for being a mediocre driver? A mediocre pilot or sailor? Of course not. The risk to life and limb would be too high. Yet, a mediocre walk carries its own health risks. It can cause physical stresses that age your body and limit your freedom of movement. You can develop chronic low back pain, stiff hips, sore knees, or stooped shoulders.

Mediocre walking can send negative signals to those who are influenced by first impressions—who are in positions to help you get promotions and better pay. You can appear uninteresting ... unsure ... sloppy ... or ... worse yet, clueless!

And how about sex appeal? A mediocre walk by implication is unsexy! Sex appeal comes from a body language that is distinctive. A woman may be naturally well endowed and look unsexy because her drab walk camouflages her physical advantages. And, the reverse is true. A woman with modest endowments may appear exciting because her walk projects vitality!

In the following pages, you learn a lot about walking. You learn why proper technique is as important to your fitness and appearance as a good pair of prescription glasses is to poor eye sight. Instruction starts with "Making a Friend of Gravity" and ends with "Heading Out, Head Held High." Along the way, you will find practicing pointers.

The process of giving yourself a walking makeover is similar to giving your face a new image. Just as you need time to feel like yourself with new makeup, you need time to adjust to moving your body in new ways.

You may find that a few of the plus+ing tips are familiar. Others may feel strange. Keep a light spirit, and practice. Once you get the feel of a Great Walk, you will get hooked and won't want to go back to your old habits.

WHEN TO PRACTICE PLUS+ING

To answer the question about when to practice, first ask yourself what kind of walker you are. Are you an on-the-job walker? A lunchtime walker? A mall walker? A club walker? A treadmill walker? A fast fitness walker who works out regularly in the early morning or evening? Perhaps you are a busy, hard-working mom who usually substitutes wheels for feet?

Fitness Walkers: If you are interested in fitness walking and have places to walk by yourself or with others on a regular basis, you can get multiple bonuses plus+ing your walk. Not only will you have a variety of things to think about and do when you are walking, you will have a new purpose for getting out the door.

The best part is that giving yourself a walking makeover can add a lot of fun to something you do anyway. Sure, it takes practice to plus your walk, but practicing takes on a new meaning when you keep your eyes on the rewards. Every time you start plus+ing some part of your walk, you are doing something special for yourself — for your fitness, appearance and life. You are making yourself a heroine in your own story.

As you will probably be using new muscles when you start plus+ing your walk, it is wise to take a gradual approach. Weak muscles will get sore if overused. For example, one day focus on your footwork and knee position. Another day practice using your hips. Another day focus on your arms and shoulders. Always pay attention to your posture.

Practice approximately one-third of your regular walking period at first. As your muscles adapt, extend the practice time until your new walk becomes your regular walk.

Roundabout Walkers If you cannot take regular fitness walks, play with the technique tips whenever you have a few moments. It isn't necessary to practice at special times, and it isn't necessary to do everything at once. Do what you can.

One young mother pluses her feet, knees and hips as she pushes her baby stroller.

Your walk can improve with short, consistent spurts of practice several times a day. In fact, practicing more than once a day grooves new moves into your motor memory more quickly than practicing one hour every so often.

•• •• WALKING WISDOM: When you plus your walk, you accomplish three goals. You benefit your health, job, and sex appeal! Who could ask for anything more?

Of course, there are more significant considerations than your walk in attaining career success and romantic fulfillment. Sense of life, ability, personality, self-esteem are just a few. Nonetheless, personal appraisals by others often start with small, subconscious and conscious observations of how you dress, how you speak, and how you walk. Why flunk any of these?

If you have always believed that walking is an ordinary skill, you should know by now that it is not. Walking is an extraordinary skill that is overlooked and underdeveloped. With this verity as your inspiration, you are now ready to start your metamorphosis.

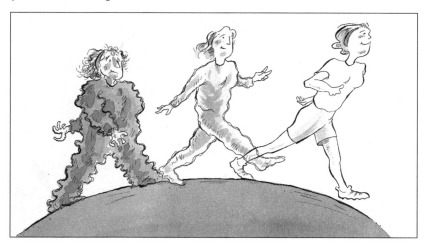

MAKING FRIENDS WITH GRAVITY

+1 POSTURE: Stand straight with your weight on the front of your feet. Head up, shoulders relaxed and chest lifted. Stomach and buttocks are tucked in. When you stand this way, you have a slight forward lean from your ankles.

Keeping your back straight and your weight on the front of your feet, lean farther and farther forward until you start falling toward the ground. BUT YOU WILL NOT FALL. Your foot will automatically reach out and save you. The force you feel pulling you down is gravity. You can make a friend of this force by maintaining a slightly forward posture as you walk. In this position, gravity pulls you ahead as you move, not down.

DYNAMIC VS STATIC

When you are standing with your weight on the front of your feet, you can bounce up and down. You are in a dynamic position ready to move. Now, rock back on your heels and try to bounce. You can't. When your weight is centered over your heels, you are in neutral, or in a static position.

Puzzlement: *If a tiger was coming at you, would you prefer to be...*
... In a static position?
... In a dynamic position?
... In an armed tank?

If you walk with a backward lean, a swayback, or a perrrfect posture, your center of gravity

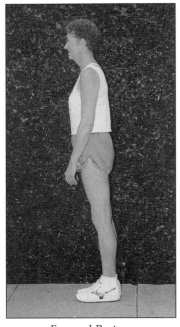

Forward Posture

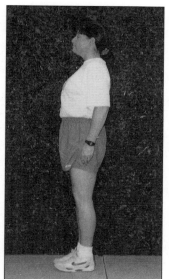

Perrrfect Posture

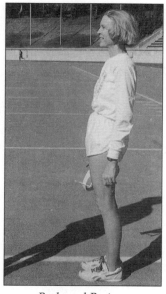

Backward Posture

goes behind or through your heels. Because gravity isn't helping you, you must generate all forward power internally.

PRACTICE POINTERS:

*** Start walking with an exaggerated backward lean and gradually come up to an erect posture. Without bending at the waist, lean forward until your nose is over your toes. When gravity starts pulling you, your feet may respond by going a bit faster.

Repeat this maneuver starting with a backward lean and gradually progressing to a forward lean. Concentrate on how the different positions feel on your feet, legs, hips and back.

When you have been walking with your weight on your heels all your life, a forward posture will feel strange but not for long. Just keep playing with it. Be sure to keep your back straight.

*** When you are outside, run a few steps. Notice how you lean forward. Most runners naturally use gravity. Now, change from running to walking. Notice whether you settle back into an erect or backward posture. Or can you keep the forward slant?

*** If you are an upright runner, shifting between running and walking won't help you. Instead, imagine that you are a Leaning Tower of Pisa moving forward.

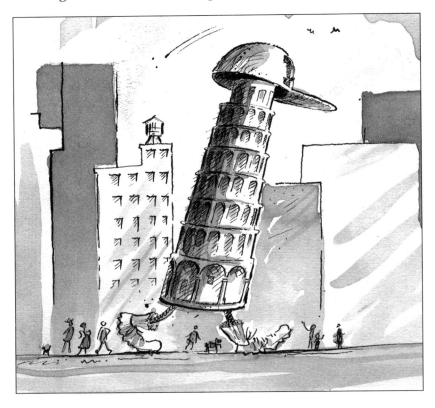

PLUS+ING BENEFITS—FORWARD POSTURE

FITNESS:

+ Making friends with gravity takes some of the work out of a workout. You are pulled forward by one of nature's strongest forces.

+ When you use gravity to walk, you can increase your speed with less effort.

+ A forward posture has proper body alignment from head to toe.

SAFETY:

+ There is safety in walking with a forward posture. Predatory men look for easy marks and usually avoid a woman who looks fit and sure of herself.

Imagine that you are leaving work late, it is dark, and the street is quite deserted. You spot a man watching you from a poorly lighted doorway, and the hair on the nape of your neck rises. You know you must not appear afraid or uncertain. If you walk with a forward, dynamic posture, you can easily and deliberately project a fit and assertive appearance. Just as importantly, you can pick up speed without revealing a burst of effort. Do not doubt your ability. Your adrenalin will pump!

APPEARANCE:

+ *Career* Visualize yourself walking toward your boss or an important customer. Picture yourself with a backward lean, a slouch, and a perrrfect posture. Now, picture yourself walking with a forward posture.

Just as leaning toward someone when you speak communicates personal interest, a forward posture conveys personal interest in meeting the person you are approaching. It aids you in establishing a context of good will. Also, it helps you project confidence in yourself and in what you are doing.

+*Romance* When you combine a forward posture with the other elements of a Great Walk, you have a walking style that is pleasing to watch. This look will be thoroughly explored and explained in the next pages.

POSTURAL PROBLEM SOLVING

Like a true friend, gravity will always be there for you when you walk, but you must meet gravity halfway. Do you have any inhibiting postural problems?

PRACTICE POINTERS:

*** If you are used to pulling your shoulders back in military style, try rounding them to bring them to neutral.

*** If you lean backward from the waist, lean forward to straighten up.

*** If you have a tendency toward a swayback, tuck in your tush and tighten your abdominal muscles.

*** If you bend forward at the waist, lift your chest up and move your shoulders back

Poor posture can be a consequence of weak or tight muscles. For example: Weak abdominal muscles and tight lower back muscles aggravate a swayback. Weak stomach and shoulder muscles aggravate a slouch. By doing strengthening and limbering exercises, you can help these problems. (See Section IV)

PUTTING YOUR FEET INTO WALKING

+2 TOES: When your toes point forward, they give purpose to your walk. Your feet look committed to the direction you are going. Straight feet also offer a boon to the lazy. Each step automatically covers maximum distance with an economy of effort.

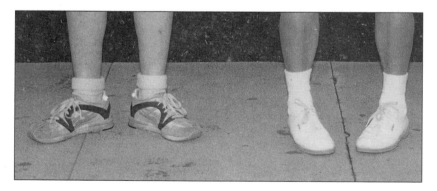

When you toe-in or toe-out, your feet are out-of-line. Wayward feet lose distance with each step. A loss of 1/2 inch every two feet amounts to a loss of 110 feet per mile.

After walking 10 miles, this loss of 1100 feet means 550 extra steps. Spread such losses out over a month, a year, a lifetime, and that's a lot of extra steps!

•● •● WALKING WISDOM: *Straight feet look neat and can't be beat.*

PLUS+ING BENEFITS – FEET POINTED FORWARD

FITNESS

+   The principal fitness benefit in walking with your feet pointed forward is body alignment. Your feet, ankles, knees and hips are properly positioned for the task of walking at any speed.

When your feet toe-out or toe-in, the alignment of your legs and hips is altered. Unnatural stress is put on the muscles and joints. This stress can cause chronic aching in seemingly remote areas of the body such as the low back, shoulders and neck.

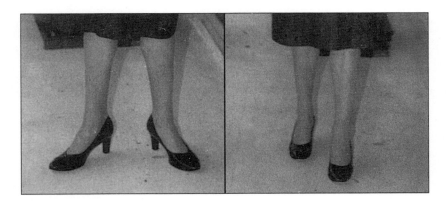

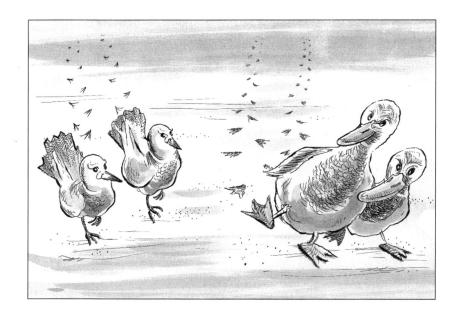

APPEARANCE

Toeing-out gives a duck-like quality to a walk. Toeing-in is frequently referred to as walking pigeon-toed and can cause a small lurching or unsteadiness. Sometimes these problems have congenital causes and cannot be helped. Much more often they are acquired habits and can be corrected. Both toeing-in and toeing-out detract from a person's overall appearance.

+ Career Close your eyes and imagine that you are selecting women to model an expensive line of suits and dresses for a hospital auxillary fashion show. One attractively dressed woman walks toward you with good posture and her toes straight forward. Another woman approaches you with knees and feet splayed out. Who is likely to get the modeling job?

+Romance If you have spent time dressing and primping to be physically attractive, be sure your feet don't sabotage your efforts. You want your feet to be flattering extensions of your legs, not at odds and angles with them.

MUCH ADO ABOUT THE HEEL

The next three plus+ing tips — heel placement, rolling and pushing — are grouped together. These tips require walking shoes with flat soles which may or may not have slightly built up heels. You will find a special tip at the end of this chapter for walking in high heels.

+3 HEEL: When your leg comes forward as you walk, raise your toes and contact the ground with your heel close to your body.

Some walkers dig their heels into the ground in front of their bodies and try to pull themselves forward. They forget that digging in is also a great way of staying put.

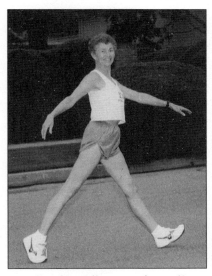

Can this walker move forward?

Forcing your foot out and pulling yourself forward with your heel is not the best way to elongate your stride, nor is it the best way to go farther, faster. Besides reducing the number of steps you can take, an extended heel acts as a slight brake, or interruption, in your stride.

PUZZLEMENT: *When your car stalls, do you get out in front and pull it? Or do you get behind and push?*

Initially, you may feel that you are taking smaller steps with a close-to-the-body heel placement, particularly if you are used to overstriding. Be reassured. Your stride may become shorter in the front, but it will compensate by getting longer in the back with the rolling and pushing tips.

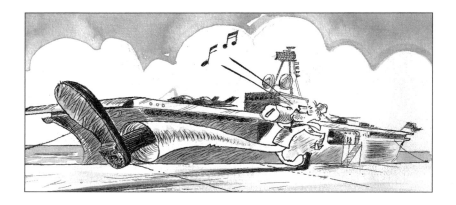

PRACTICE POINTERS:

As the footwork starts with correct heel placement, you need to become aware of your heel contacting the ground.
*** Walk on your heels with your legs straight.

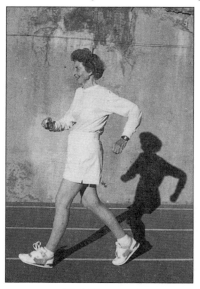

Heel Placement

*** Stand and put your weight on your left foot. Raise your right foot off the ground and come down on the back edge of your heel. Repeat this move several times. Switch sides.
*** When you are walking, imagine that you have a metal tap on the back of the heel of your shoe. Focus on contacting the ground on this imaginary tap. If you listen to music with a headset, you can synchronize the beat of the music to the "tapping" of your heel. Music can help you feel rhythm.

ROLL, ROLL, ROLL

+4 THE ROLL: Start walking. After contacting the ground with your heel and toes up, roll forward along the outer, fleshy surface of your sole. By keeping your heel contact close to your body, you can roll forward in an uninterrupted, continuous motion.

If you are not certain where to roll, look at the bottom of one of your feet. On the inside, you will see a depression where your arch is. Toward the outside, you will see a smooth surface extending from heel to toe. This surface is the natural pathway for rolling.

PRACTICE POINTERS:

*** Pretend that your right foot is a rocker on a rocking chair. Keeping your right leg straight, rock forward from heel to toe and backward from toe to heel. Now, rock with your left foot. Practice until the rocking or rolling motion feels easy with both feet.

*** Taking very small steps, come down on the back part of your heel and roll up to your tiptoes with one foot and then the other. Walk this way until your leg muscles start getting tired, which may be fairly quickly. The objective is to gain control of the heel-to-toe roll. Repeat this footwork each time you go walking. You'll improve the strength in your legs and ankles as you do it.

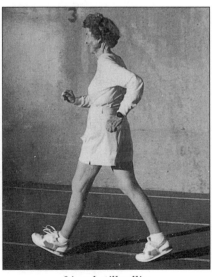

84 and still rolling

PUSHING POWER

+5 THE PUSH: To give more power to your walk, combine rolling with pushing. Roll forward and as your foot passes under you, gently push the ground back. If you have to get somewhere in a hurry, push harder with the front of your foot and the pads of your toes.

You will be surprised how tough your toes are when asked to work. You will also be surprised how pushing increases the length of your stride.

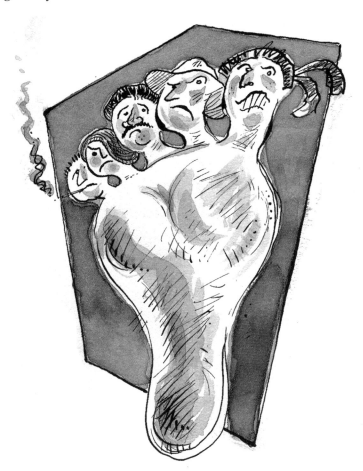

PRACTICE POINTERS:

*** Play with massaging the ground from heel to toe along the fleshy surface of your sole.

*** Play with pushing the ground back with the front of your foot and the pads of your toes.

***Then roll—push, roll—push, roll—push merrily along the road.

•• •• *WALKING WISDOM: When you put your feet into walking, you make a partner of the ground.*

SUMMARY +3, +4, +5

• As your foot comes forward, raise your toes and contact the ground toward the back edge of your heel.

• Heel contact is close to your body.

• Roll forward from heel to toe on the fleshy surface of the sole of your foot.

• As your foot passes to the rear, push the ground back for extra power.

PLUS+ING BENEFITS — FOOT USE

FITNESS

+ It takes strength to flex the ankles and raise your toes in the air. Developing this ability as you walk will overcome weakness and instability in your ankles.

+ Flexing your ankle to raise your toes stretches your back leg muscles and prevents these muscles from contracting and contributing to an "old" looking, bent-knee walk.

+ Ankle flexing to raise your toes also helps slim and shape your calves far more successfully than walking with a flat-footed stride.

+ By using your foot from heel to toe, you can stimulate the circulation in your feet. Better circulation can help cold feet as well as ankle edema.

+ The combination of the gentle tapping of your heels on the ground and the rolling motion of your feet gives a rhythmic, gliding quality to your walk. This gait feels good any time. It can feel especially soothing when you are worried, anxious or depressed.

+ If you add pushing to your footwork, you will find additional comfort. Just as hitting a tennis ball hard or pounding a pillow can release anger and frustration, so can pushing the ground back vigorously with each step.

SAFETY

+ There is an important safety benefit in raising your toes and rolling from heel to toe. If you decide you want to walk more briskly, rolling minimizes the impact of your foot on the ground. It prevents the front of your foot from slapping the hard surface and jarring your ankles, knees and lower back as often happens in faster flatfooted walking.

Rolling also can help prevent blisters from friction and black toe from hitting the toe box, especially when you are walking downhill.

APPEARANCE

+ *Career* On occasions, you may feel pressured at work and be tense and tired. You need a practical antidote to boss or client stress. A few minutes of deep breathing or meditation can help; so can walking.

A lunch hour walk, even a short one, can help mend the tatters of mind and spirit. Focus on using the rolling, pushing footwork and on feeling its rhythm.

+ *Romance* Visualize this scene. Your church is sponsoring a fund-raising walk for a charity. You are new to the congregation and decide it would be a good way to meet people. You start out walking with a woman in her late fifties whose walk appears smooth and effortless, even though she is going at a quick pace. Wanting to keep up with her, you find yourself taking big steps and big arm swings, and soon feel perspiration running down your back. After a mile, you find an excuse to join a man you met briefly the previous Sunday. As you walk up to him, you have a momentary wish that you could walk like the woman you just left.

HIGH HEELS

High heels are for vanity. They are flattering to the legs and figure, and complement dresses, suits and evening clothes. When you wear high heels, your weight is tipped toward your toes. Because this weight distribution puts unnatural stress on your ankles, legs, hips and back, it is wise to limit their use if you have any problems with these areas. With this said, let's be real. Although low heels or walking shoes are sensible, they don't take the place of pretty shoes.

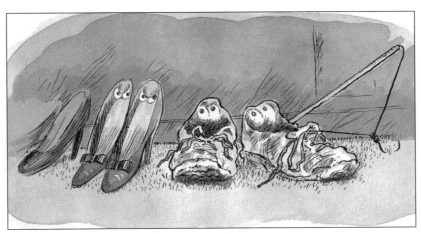

+ HIGH HEELS: When you are walking, high heeled shoes help you hold a forward posture, but they inhibit you from raising your toes. Therefore, bring your heel down under your body with toes pointed forward. Gently push the ground behind you with the front of your foot. This pushing opens your stride in the back and will stimulate a natural hip movement.

You will never feel slightly awkward or ungainly wearing heels if you follow this special tip. The close-to-the-body heel placement, straight ahead toes, and gentle pushing of the ground lead to a fluid, smooth gait that truly complements your appearance.

RESPECTING YOUR NOBLE KNEE

KNEES WITH CLASS

What is the best-kept walking secret?

A bent-knee walk is not attractive. Carried to the extreme, it looks funny. Remember Groucho Marx's exaggerated, semi-crouching walk?

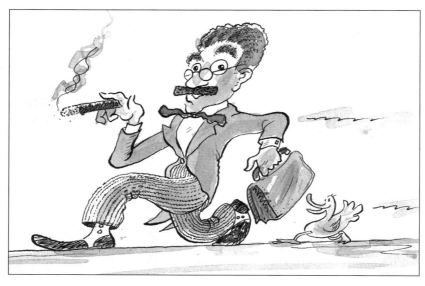

If you walk with bent knees, no one will laugh or turn away. But, take a hint. Do yourself a favor and try unbending!

If you want an attractive walk, you want your knees to give a clean, sharp line to your legs and a confident, smooth quality to your stride. You want knees that straighten in the vertical, support position.

It doesn't matter what type of build you have or whether you have extra pounds. A straight supporting leg adds style to your walk.

Some women naturally walk with their legs straight in the support position. A much larger group do not. If you are a bent-knee walker, it may take you a while to get your knee to straighten, but YOU'RE WORTH IT!

STRAIGHT IS COOL

+6 KNEE STRAIGHTENING:

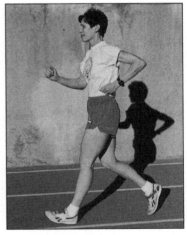

Straight leg

Start walking. Straighten your knee as you raise your toes during the forward phase of your leg swing. After heel contact with the ground, keep your leg straight, or as straight as you can, into the support position.

🏃 *Getting to know the muscles that straighten and bend your knee:*

QUADRICEPS: The muscles above your knees in the front of your thighs are your quadriceps. The "quads" consist of four separate muscles, and they are responsible for straightening your knees.

To feel your quadriceps working, put your hands on your thighs just above your knee caps. Do a shallow knee bend. As you unbend, you will feel your quadriceps harden as they contract to straighten your knees.

A quadriceps muscle of special interest is the vastus medialis. This little muscle helps straighten the knee the last 15 degrees. The vastus medialis is located just above and to the inside of your knee cap. In the past, you may well have had some kind of knee or leg injuries, or worn ill-fitting shoes that caused you to limp or walk abnormally. If so, did you notice that your quads got weak quickly? The vastus medialis was the first to go. Unless you made a point of rehabilitating this muscle with specific exercises, it may not have regained its original strength and may be less effective in stabilizing and straightening your knee now.

HAMSTRINGS: The muscles in the back of your thighs are called the hamstrings. They are responsible for bending your knees. When you bend your knees, the hamstrings contract, and when you straighten your knees, they stretch.

To feel the action in your hamstrings, sit in a chair and put your right hand on the hamstrings of your right leg. Bend and straighten your knee to feel your hamstrings contract and stretch. If you can reach down to your calf muscles, you will feel these muscles contract and extend with the bending and straightening of your knee.

It is quite common for the hamstrings and other back leg muscles to shorten with advancing years. If this has happened to you, your knees may be quite set in a bent position; and, like it or not, you may have to walk with bent legs. Raising your toes as you walk helps keep the back leg muscles stretched and youthful.

If you cannot walk with straight knees, you will find helpful strengtheners for your quadriceps as well as stretches for your hamstrings and calves in Section Four.

NO FORCE, PLEASE

+7 KNEE SAFETY:

Straightening the knee does not refer to "locking" or "forcing" the knee straight by pulling with the heel. Heel contact should never involve any pulling. When your toes are up and your heel contacts the ground close to your body, you can straighten your knee without harmful stress.

If you walk with bent knees, making the effort to develop knee awareness may be all that is required to change your habit. If you naturally straighten your knees as you walk, do these practice pointers just to feel the difference between straight-knee walking and bent-knee walking.

PRACTICE POINTERS:

*** Standing in front of a mirror, watch yourself slowly bend and straighten your knees. Now, close your eyes and do more knee bends. As you straighten your legs, feeeeel your knees straighten.

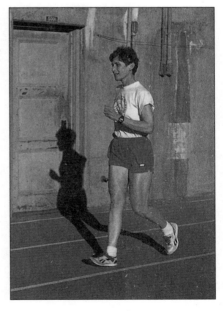

*** If you walk with bent knees, become aware of how bent-knee walking feels by exaggerating like Groucho.

*** Walk slowly and deliberately straighten your legs before heel contact. Don't think about it too much. Just do it! Flexing your ankles and raising your toes high helps.

*** Walk on your heels with your legs straight.

*** Taking very small steps, contact the ground with the

Knee safety

edge of your heel and your leg straight. Roll forward keeping your leg straight into the vertical support position. By taking small steps, you can better control the straightening process of your knees.

REMINDER: You know how to walk. Plus+ing your knee only refers to having a straight knee when your leg is under you. Your knee quite properly bends as your foot leaves the ground and swings forward. The straightening process begins just before heel contact when you flex your ankle to bring your toes up. Play with plus+ing your knee. Your walk deserves a royal flair, and once you get it, you'll like it.

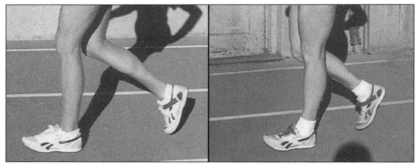

Bent knee   Straight knee

PLUS+ING BENEFITS – STRAIGHT KNEE

FITNESS

+ When your knee is straight in the support position, your body weight is carried by your leg bones, the femur, tibia, and fibula. When your knee is bent, the muscles around your knee must support your weight. As muscles tire, using the bones for support adds stability and endurance to your walking.

+ A straight leg provides firm support for a smooth, heel-toe roll at all speeds.

+ Because exercise striders and power walkers often walk with very bent knees, their energy goes in three directions: up, down and forward. Given that their goal is moving forward, the up/down motions are counterproductive and inefficient. When your knee straightens in the support position, up/down movement is reduced. If your posture has a forward lean as well, it is practically eliminated.

APPEARANCE

+ *Career* Imagine yourself arriving at a job interview. You know that there are several other qualified people applying for the same position. You want to project confidence in your job qualifications, as you feel a great opportunity awaits if you can "put it all together". You enter a room with the person in charge looking you over. Do you walk with knees that give a refined line to your leg and a lift to your appearance? Or do you walk with knees that sag?

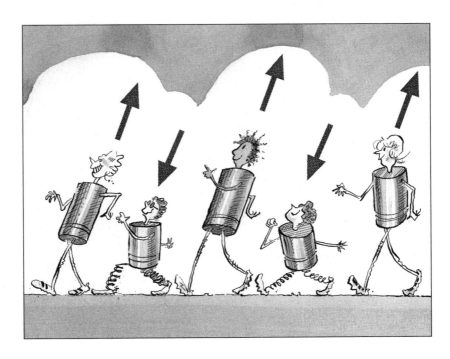

+ Romance You are in your car waiting for the red light to change. You watch two men crossing the street in front of you. Both are well built and have nice faces, but they do zero for you. You notice that they are striding with very bent legs, and you suddenly realize, "What a difference a knee makes."

GETTING HIP TO YOUR HIPS

HIP HANG-UPS

Hips have a hard time in our society. From childhood on we've been warned to avoid wiggling, waggling, sashaying, bumping and grinding. Given so many don'ts, it's not surprising that using the hips in walking provokes a smirk, a frown or jeer from many men and women.

• Does the idea of using your hips when you walk bother you?

• Do you think rotating your hips looks provocative?

• Do you worry that rotating your hips will hurt your lower back?

• Do you think a man looks swishy or effeminate if he uses his hips walking?

These are questions that reflect a common concern among many women and men.

𐀏Getting to know your hips:

HIP JOINT: The hip joint connects the upper leg bone (femur) to the pelvis; the term "hip" refers to the area surrounding the hip joint and lateral to it — including the fleshy part of the upper thigh. The hip joint is a ball and socket and has an extensive range of motion. In walking, it allows the leg to swing forward and backward.

PELVIS: The pelvis is the big bony encasement at the lower end of the trunk below your waist. It supports the spine. The lower back joints make it possible to rotate the pelvis and hips.

HIP ROTATION: The hip movement that needs to be freed of silly sexual overtones in walking is pelvic-hip rotation. As discussed earlier, in a natural walk, the pelvis and hips rotate together with the forward and backward movement of the legs. Hip rotation automatically involves pelvic rotation. 🚶

IT'S NOT ABOUT SEX!

Kissing happens to involve the mouth, but we don't consider all uses of the mouth sexy. We use our mouths in many activities. We talk, we eat, and sometimes we whistle.

Making love happens to involve the hips, but we don't consider all uses of the hips sexy. We use them in many different sports and social activities. Watch soccer players, swimmers or dancers.

Tell a group of children that there is ice cream on the other side of a swimming pool; then tell them that they must walk to get it. You will see a spontaneous demonstration of hip rotation as they race each other.

By deliberately restricting the rotation of the hips, walkers arrest the flow of movement in their bodies. They also effectively isolate their arms and legs in two zones.

The Tin Man in the Wizard of Oz is a figure with arms and legs attached to a rigid, metal body. You can see many tin men and tin women walking on the streets. All that's missing is the grating "clank" and "boink.

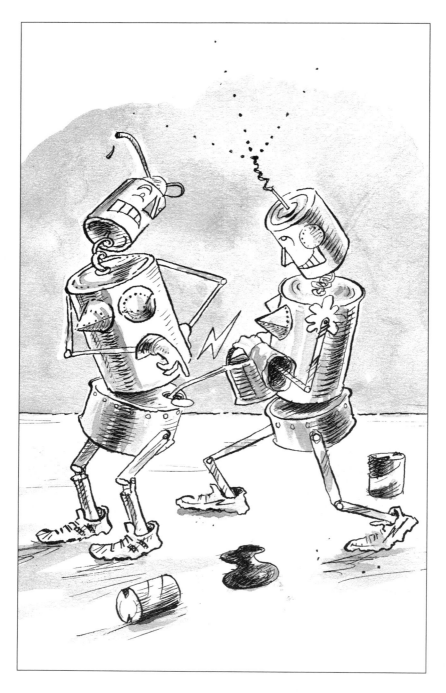

NATURAL HIP ROTATION

+8 HIPS: When you walk, let your hips rotate forward as your leg swings forward and backward as your leg goes behind you. The rotation is maximally forward when your heel contacts the ground, and maximally backward as your toes leave the ground. There is no "boomteeay" or sashay. No side-to-side sway or gyration. You will feel a twisting at your waist as your hips rotate.

If the movements of your hips and legs are already in sync, you have an advantage. On the other hand, if you do not rotate your hips when you walk, it may take a little practice and a little good-humored patience to get them going. When you get it right, you'll know it.

PRACTICE POINTERS:

*** With your arms akimbo, turn or rotate your pelvis backward and forward smoothly and evenly so you can feel your waist twisting. Do not turn your shoulders. Keep your shoulders on a frontal plane and still.

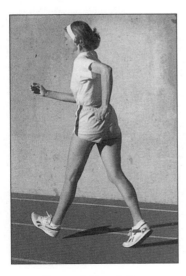

Forward hip rotation

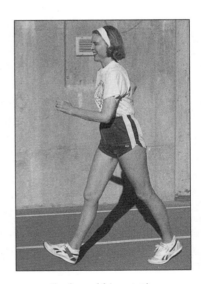

Backward hip rotation

*** Chubby Checkers and "The Twist" were a Sixties craze. If you know how, try "doin' the twist". See and feel your hips "twisting" back and forth.

*** Start walking and imagine that your leg extends to your waist. To use this longer leg, you must rotate your hips by relaxing and moving your hips forward and backward with your legs. Keep thinking about walking from your waist. It is not unusual to get the rotation going and then to lose it. Gradually, you will be able to sustain the rotation for longer and longer periods until it goes on autopilot.

*** As you are walking, check on whether you feel twisting in your waist. If you don't feel the twisting, you will know you have stopped rotating your hips.

PLUS+ING BENEFITS – HIP ROTATION

FITNESS

+ Rotating your hips as you walk is a sure way of trimming your waistline and surrounding areas. Try to walk this way at all times. If you watch your diet as well, your extra fat is doomed. Keep a tape measure handy!

+ A gentle, steady hip rotation massages the lower back muscles and can alleviate spasm and pain. It also can keep the back limber to counter the stiffening process of arthritis and aging. If you add the abdominal and lower back plus+ers in Section IV, you may even enjoy freedom from pain.

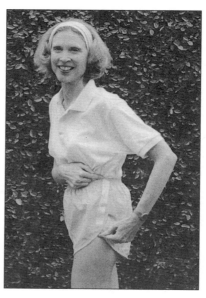

Adding inches to stride

+ The best way of elongating your stride is to add hip rotation to your walk. If you do not add this rotation, the length of your stride is limited by the length of your legs. By utilizing the span between the top of your leg and your waist, you add several inches to your stride. Competitive racewalkers add five to six inches by using a complete forward and backward rotation.

APPEARANCE

+ Career Tonight, when you go to bed try this mental role playing. You have been promoted to a management level position and will be involved with meeting people important to the company and to your job success. Visualize yourself walking to meet a VIP with toes pointing forward, legs straightening and hips rotating easily. Now visualize yourself toeing out, knees bent, and a motionless trunk.

By making hip rotation a natural part of your walk, the movements of your upper body and lower body coordinate. The resulting walk looks supple and communicates positive energy. On the other hand, a duckfooted, bent-knee walk with little upper body motion is very ordinary. It does not give you any first impression advantage.

+ Romance: Because you may have some inhibitions about letting your hips rotate when you walk, let's explore this reluctance.

From the burlesque bump-and-grinders to Elvis and the hard rock stars, pelvic gyrations and thrusts have been part of our musical pop culture. Performers have meant these movements to be associated with sexuality, and their audiences have been accepting.

In a plus+ed walk, hip rotation is related to the forward and backward movement of the legs. Its purpose is to increase stride length and to integrate the body's movements.

The effects of hip rotation on a woman's walk and appearance are essentially pleasing and, consequently, contribute to her attractiveness. For example, let's consider the legs. If you rotate your hips, your legs look longer regardless of what you are wearing. Many women want long legs because many men consider long legs "sexy".

Secondly, a smooth hip rotation allows you to combine your walking movements so that your body moves as a whole, rather than in parts. This coordination can give your walk a special rhythm and vitality that sparks attention. Ask most men if they aren't attracted to a woman who uses her body well when she walks.

Moving your hips as a natural extension of moving your legs injects energy into your whole body's dynamics. It contributes to your sex appeal without requiring any overt sexual display. If you have any doubt, role-play once more.

Imagine that you are entering a party and see "him" across a room. You would like "him" to notice you. How do you want to appear to him? Do you want to look fit and natural, or tight and reserved? Which "you" do you think would attract "him"?

Don't be reluctant to rotate your hips when you walk. Hip rotation does not have to be exaggerated. Less than one-half inch of movement delivers desirable fitness and appearance benefits. Cast doubt aside. Have fun. Be natural. Free your hips, free your walk and enjoy knowing that your body looks good in motion.

PEOPLE-WATCHING

This is a good time for another field trip to a busy downtown corner or shopping mall. Find a good observation point and study how women and men treat their hips. Out of ten walkers, how many use their hips when they walk? Do you see twisting motion at their waists?

You may see some women with a deliberate side-to-side tush swing. You may also notice that some men overstride as a substitute for using their hips. Studying how people use and misuse their bodies can highlight the advantages in plus+ing your walk.

MAKING YOUR ARMS PART OF THE ACTION

COMPATIBLE ARMS

When you are walking, the direction of your arm swing is important. As you walk from your car to the market, or from your desk to the fax machine, do your arms cooperate? If they swing back and forth symmetrically at your sides, they fulfill their supporting role. Their energy augments the energy of your legs.

When Ginger Rogers and Fred Astaire danced, their movements looked effortless because their teamwork was complete. Neither would have allowed their arms or legs to move in conflicting directions. No matter how difficult the choreography, they moved as one.

ARMED CONFLICT

If your arms swing across your body, they cause your hips to move from side to side. In effect, your arms and hips *move* in one direction (sideways) and your legs *move* in another direction (forward).

The same conflict is created when you force your arms to swing very high in front or high in back, as in power walking. The upward momentum of your arms lifts your body while your legs work to go forward.

Consider a police officer telling you to go left with one hand and to go straight with the other. You probably would feel quite confused until you received a clear message on how to proceed.

WALKING WISDOM: *The legs of four-legged animals move forward and backward. Human arms and legs should move forward and backward, too. If you are uncertain about this, picture a horse walking with one front foot going sideways.*

THE SWING

+9 LONG ARM SWING: Start walking. Keeping your shoulders relaxed, let your arms swing symmetrically back and forth at your sides. Hands are relaxed with fingers slightly curled. Palms face in.

+10 SHORTENED ARM SWING: For fitness walking, bend your elbows to form an 85 to 90 degree angle. When your arms swing backward, bring your wrists just behind your buttocks. When your arms swing forward, bring your elbows to the middle of your sides. Keep your hands below midchest.

Hold your hands in loose fists with your thumbs resting lightly on your index fingers. To add style, slightly cock your wrist. A hand that dangles down from a limp wrist looks geekish.

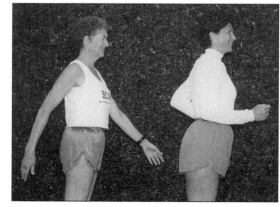

SIZING THE SWING

+11 **SWING & STRIDE LENGTH:** The size of your arm swing influences the length of your stride. Start walking, but barely move your arms. Note the length of your stride. Swing your arms in a moderate arc. Again, note the length of your stride. Finally, note the length of your stride when you swing your arms fully.

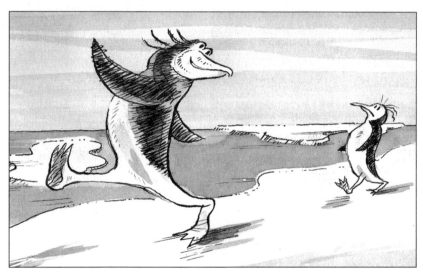

• A full arm swing promotes a full stride.
• A medium arm swing promotes a medium stride.
• Little-to-no arm swing promotes .....
...The two penguins know!

Many fitness walkers keep their entire arm swing in front of their bodies which tends to restrict hip movement. A full swing helps you rotate your hips.

DON'TS
• Don't swing one or both arms across your body.
• Don't pump your arms high in front or high in back.

•Don't punch the air or make a circular motion in front of your body when your arms are bent at the elbows.

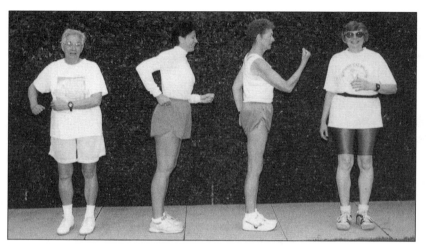

| Arms swinging across | Swing too high in back | Swing too high in front | Swinging in different directions |

PRACTICE POINTERS:

Using your arms correctly for regular walking and for fitness walking is easy to do. However, bad habits can interfere. If one of your arms goes forward and back and the other goes across your body, you may have trouble retraining the crossing arm. Even small changes need time to imprint on your motor memory.

Concentrate on altering an errant arm swing as if you were learning the scales on a piano. Only after you have truly focused on practicing the scales without errors does the fingering become automatic. The same focus is needed to adjust your arms to swing properly.

FOR LONG ARMS

Standing in front of a mirror, and then walking...

*** Swing your arms back and forth at your sides.

*** Swing your arms across your body (with elbows going out).

*** Swing one arm back and forth, and one across. Feel the effects on your lower back.

FOR SHORT ARMS

*** Stand sideways in front of a mirror so you can look at your right arm hanging down. Now, bend your right elbow in a 90 degree angle, and touch your elbow to your side. With your left index finger, draw a line from back to front through the point where your elbow touches. The line is parallel to the ground. It may be at, above, or below your waist, depending on the length of your upper arm from shoulder to elbow. Your shortened arm should swing along this line. Your left arm will have a similar swing line.

*** Continue standing side ways before a mirror with your right arm bent at the elbow. Keeping your shoulder relaxed, start swinging your arm. Swing your arm backward so your wrist goes just behind your buttocks and forward so your elbow comes to the middle of your side. Think elbow-wrist, elbow-wrist as you watch your elbow and wrist moving back and forth along your natural swing line.

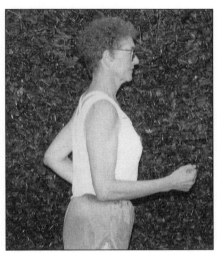

Short arm swing line

*** Stand facing a mirror. Thrust your hands way up in front and your elbows way up in back as in power walking. See and feel your body lifting. Return to an efficient, easy back and forth movement, always keeping your hands below midchest.

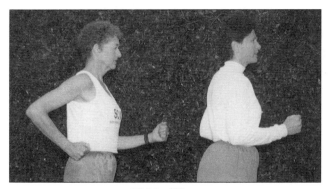

Wrist - Elbow

WALKING ARM SWING

*** While walking, experiment with all of the long and short arm combinations. Try walking fast with long and short arms. Isn't it easier and much more comfortable to walk fast with your arms short? Be sure to check that your arms swing behind you, not just in front. A full back swing assists a forward posture.

REMINDERS - SHORTENED ARMS:
 Think elbow-wrist.
 Move arms along natural swing lines.
 Keep hands below mid chest.

PLUS+ING BENEFITS - ARM SWING

FITNESS

+ If you bend your elbows in a 90 degree angle to shorten your arms, you can walk faster. A long arm, like a long pendulum, moves more slowly and acts as a drag on faster paces. A shortened arm, like a short pendulum, moves more quickly.

+   When your shortened arms swing in natural, contained arcs, their regular back and forth movement massages and soothes sore, tight shoulder and neck muscles.

+   A shortened arm swing is also a cure for "fat fingers."

Some walkers find that their fingers swell when they have been walking for a long time with their arms hanging down. Body fluids pool in the hands causing the fingers to fatten. If you have this problem, try walking with a shortened arm swing to get relief.

APPEARANCE

+ *Career and Romance:* Few people truly coordinate the movements of their arms, hips and legs. Arms that swing across the stomach or that go in contrary directions look awkward; but they, too, are a very common sight. No one will point a finger at you if your arms go in different directions. At the same time, no one will take notice of you either. You simply blend in with the other average pedestrians.

When you synchronize your arms with the forward movements of your legs and body, your walk takes on the aura of Grrrreatness. Just like a cool breeze feels good on a warm day, a fully-coordinated walk feels good and looks good all the time. You will enjoy a sense of inner assurance when you enter your boss' office, take a customer to luncheon, or walk down the street with a colleague. You will know that your walking appearance is a career asset to you.

What applies to your career, applies to your social life. Most men are stimulated by what they see. Be sure to give the man you want to attract a walk that is worth watching. You will have a jump-start on romance.

HEADING OUT, HEAD HELD HIGH CREATING AN ATTITUDE

+12 THE HEAD: Head up! Eyes forward! That's the attitude of a Great Walk. You want to look like you want to go wherever you are going.

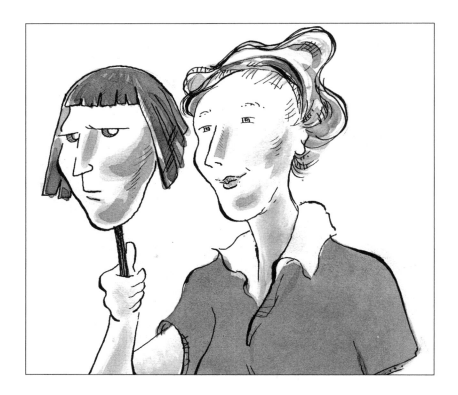

If along the way you meet people and it seems appropriate, smile. Smiling is a muscle relaxant. It relaxes your face, chin and neck muscles when you are anxious and tense. When an open smile may not be wise, smile inwardly. An inner smile has the same calming effect.

•● ●● WALKING WISDOM: *You always want to walk like you have the world by the tail.*

PRACTICE POINTERS

*** Deliberately bend your neck to look down at your feet. Feel how the heavy weight of your head stresses your neck, shoulder and back muscles. As you bring your head up into alignment, feel these muscles relax.

Your head is like a 17-pound bowling ball centered on the neck of a bowling pin. When your head is in alignment, it requires little muscle strength to hold it in position. As your head falls away from the vertical, it requires greater and greater muscle strength to hold it up. Another reason for neck and shoulder muscle tension.

*** If you have a habit of looking down at the ground when you walk, lower your eyes instead of bending your head.

*** A way of reminding yourself to keep your head up is to select objects that are eye level or a little higher as check points.

*** Adjusting the angle of your head for a sideways tilt is easier said than done. It requires "proprioception"—getting the feel of holding your head erect and of being able to sense when it is not.

*** If you look in a mirror and can see that your neck and head project forward from your shoulders, you are developing a road runner's neck. It is difficult to correct this abnormal position, though limbering exercises can help some. Be warned. Pull your head back in while you can.

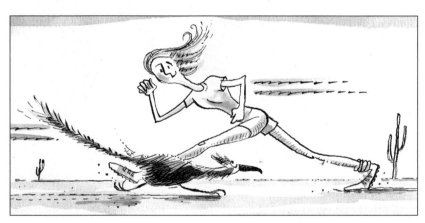

PLUS+ING BENEFITS – HEAD UP

FITNESS

+   When your head is up and in alignment with your spine, your neck, shoulder and upper back muscles can stay relaxed.
+   Balance and coordination also improve when the head is properly positioned.

SAFETY

+   A head-up, in-control attitude is another way of giving potential molesters second thoughts. Imagine that you are taking a walk in your neighborhood at dawn. You seldom feel anxious walking alone, but the news has been filled with the rape of a woman who lives a few blocks away.

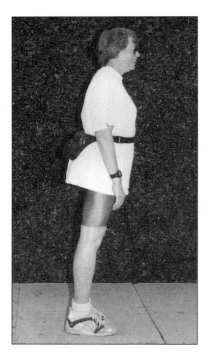

You decide to go back home. You continue walking at the same brisk pace, hiding your feelings of vulnerability. Your posture is forward, your head is up and your face appears calm, but determined. You want to look in-charge, not like an easy victim.

APPEARANCE

+ *Career and Romance:* When your head is up, you can convey a positive attitude about who you are and what you are doing. You know from your own experience that when others walk with assurance, you see and feel it; and when they face you openly and pleasantly, you are more apt to feel friendly. You can use such body language whenever you walk.

For example, in your relationships with men and women who influence your financial security and career success, be sure to keep your head up and your eyes amiable in your meetings and greetings. You will appear to be comfortable and confident to them. They will feel that you are secure about yourself. This type of self-affirming message does not preclude showing respect. It simply means holding your head with poise to let significant others feel that you have faith in yourself and in your abilities.

Keeping your head up is also a wise defense to life's downers and a smart offense to life's challenges. When you are feeling discouraged and would prefer crawling into a dark hole to going to work some morning, force yourself out the door with your head up. After a few steps, stop and take a deep breath. Then, proceed. By looking straight out at the world, you can better reassert your value to yourself — an important strategy of successful women.

There are times for pain and suffering, and it's dumb to pretend otherwise. There are also times when the best cure for problems is to head toward your goals. Holding your head high when you walk helps you feel that you can overcome disappointments and loss. It also can help you cope with others' irrational behavior. Never let others make you feel "lesser than" they. Be a Great Walker and keep your HEAD UP!

SECRETS OF A GREAT WALK

Posture: A Great Walk has a slight forward lean to make a friend of gravity.

Feet: A Great Walk has forward pointing toes, a close-to-the-body heel placement and a rolling, pushing rhythm from heel to toe.

Knees: A Great Walk has straight knees in the support position.

Hips: A Great Walk has an easy, forward and backward hip rotation.

Arms: A Great Walk has an efficient, economical arm swing that mirrors the forward and backward movement of the legs, whether the arms are long for regular walking or shortened for fitness walking.

Head: A Great Walk is always, "Head Up!"

When you walk with a forward posture and with the other elements of the plus+ing technique, you will have a Great Walk. Your footwork will have rhythm; your knees will give your legs a clean, uplifting line; your hips will integrate the movements of your upper body and lower body; your arms will provide coordination; and your head will make a leading statement. You will have every reason to feel good about your walking appearance and to know that others will feel good about it too.

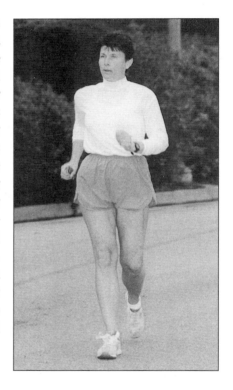

•● •● **WALKING WISDOM: Nature's walking plan is very simple. All systems forward.**

PRACTICING POST-TIPS

♩ MAKE IT MUSICAL

When you are practicing the 12 plus+ing tips, think of the music you like, or better yet, get a headset. Music will help you get rhythm in your footwork. It also will help you blend

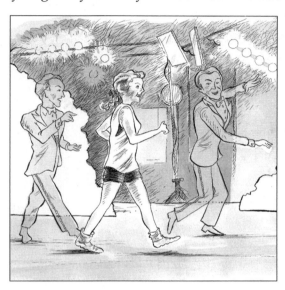

the movements of your legs, hips and arms. (When wearing a headset, always keep the volume down so that you can hear the noises around you. Alternatively, you can move the earphones in front of your ear canals and have the volume louder. This forward position will protect your eardrums from the pounding of a closed vacuum system.)

As you improve your heel-toe roll and as you feel your body moving in unity, you will experience a sense of wonderful lightness and flow which is akin to dancing.

👁 VISUALIZATION

What you see in your mind's eye can influence your actions because your central nervous system does not know the difference between imagined and real events. This curious fact makes it possible for you to practice plus+ing techniques in your imagination as well as in reality.

To try visualization, make use of 10 or 15 minutes of quiet time. Close your eyes and see yourself with a Great Walk.

Rehearse the technique tips as if you were in fact practicing them. See yourself moving with gravity. Feel the air about you, the wind in your hair, the warmth of the sun on your body. See your feet, legs, hips and arms working evenly and symmetrically together. Feel the gentle tapping of your heel at ground contact, and feel your feet rolling smoothly under you. Literally participate in an inner motion picture of yourself.

Mary Lou Retton, Greg Louganis and many other Olympians visualized all facets of their techniques before their medal-winning performances. Mary Lou visualized all her gymnastic routines the night before competition. Greg used visualization between dives, and again when he stood on the diving board or platform before performing. These extraordinary athletes have stated that mental rehearsal was a key to their success.

Try visualization. It works. It makes adopting new walking habits easier.

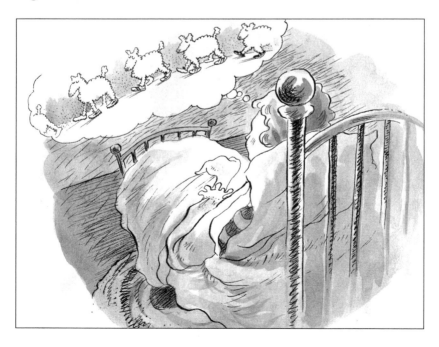

PLUS+ERS

*Giving
Extra Wow
to
Your Walk*

୨ଚ

PLUS+ERS

A Great Walk has a special style that is reinforced by flex-ibility. A flexible body walks easily and does not tire quickly. The range of motion in the joints is full, and the muscles are limber. In contrast, tight muscles, like chains, set confining limits on what your body can do. They can restrict the pleas-ure you enjoy in walking.

A Great Walk has a special strength. Strong muscles make it possible to project energy and vitality into a walk. They support confident, attractive movement. In contrast, weak muscles can lead to a slouching, uninteresting, sexless walk.

In this section, you are introduced to carefully selected mobility plus+ers. Each plus+er affects the strength and/or flexibility of specific muscles or joints in your body. Approach them as you would a winning lottery ticket or an aphrodisiac. They can add extra "wow" to your walk.

THE FOUR S's

Increasing mobility not only involves Stretching and Strengthening, it also involves Smiling. You will quickly understand the need for a sense of humor when you are stand-ing next to someone who can bend over like a piece of spaghet-ti while you struggle to bend a few inches. Success in stretch-ing comes with a inner chuckle, not just with performance.

One of the best by-products of mobility is a fourth "S": Spontaneity. By increasing strength along with flexibility, you can regain some of that marvelous nimble quality of a child. In a word, you can reinvent the stereotype of aging.

So be patient and persist. As with many things of value, mobility comes gradually to some of us.

•• •• WALKING WISDOM: An "old" walk is stiff. A "young" walk is mobile. There are no age limits.

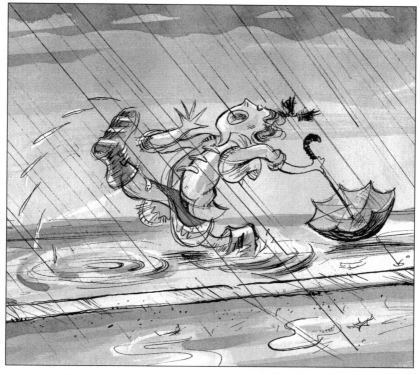

A 20-year-old girl can have stiff joints and weak muscles. A 75-year-old woman can have limber joints and strong muscles. These mobility truths have scrambled relationships between men and women. It is no longer unusual to see older, fit women attracting younger men. Not only do these sirens have youthful strength and flexibility, they have mental maturity. A winning combination.

SOME COMMON SENSE

As you try the different mobility plus+ers, be sure to pay heed to any injury, arthritis or other physical problems you may have. Always consult a doctor if in doubt. These plus+ers will be beneficial in limbering and strengthening problem areas, but never persist if you feel pain. A little discomfort when you stretch tight muscles is okay, but pain is not okay. Similarly, a little soreness when you strengthen weak muscles is all right, but pain is not. Persisting pain is a sign you have done too much. Ease up.

Your body is your playmate. Plus+ing your walk means plus+ing your body as it is — imperfections and all. As with the technique tips, if you are unable to do some of the suggested stretches or strengtheners, fine. Do what you can do. The goal is to increase your rewards in walking.

PLUS+ER POINTERS

*** Whenever you bend or straighten a body part such as an arm or leg, you stretch and strengthen opposing muscle groups. A simple movement does both.

*** Plus+ers are good for rehabilitating joints and muscles as well as for preventing injury.

*** Most women have weak ankles because they have knowingly or unknowingly sustained sprains at least once in their lives. Ankle plus+ers not only will help you strengthen the muscles around your ankles, they will energize your walk.

*** Plus+ers for straightening your knees can alleviate some minor pains and chronic problems by developing strength and stability in the support structures.

*** To move your hips easily, it is necessary to have limber back and side muscles. By doing the hip plus+ers regularly, you may start to notice a definite improvement in the way your body feels and moves within a few weeks.

*** For your arms to complement the movement of your legs, your shoulders need to be flexible. Shoulder plus+ers are range of motion maneuvers. They can be good substitutes for aspirin when your shoulders, neck and head ache from tension.

HOW MUCH,
HOW OFTEN:

Try all of the plus+ers, if you can, over a couple of weeks. Find those you like the best. When you have picked your favorites, settle on a convenient and comfortable time of day or night to do them regularly for 10 to 15 minutes. Three times a week is okay. Six to seven times a week is outstanding.

Stretches: Hold every stretch at least 15 seconds, preferably 20 to 30 seconds. There has been some experimentation in having elite competitive athletes hold stretches 3 and 4 minutes. This is not necessary for you.

Strengtheners: Increase the number of strengtheners you do gradually to avoid sore muscles. However, remember you are not a machine that gradually revs up as you get into condition. You will have up days and down days. The trend should be to increase the strengtheners until you have reached an effective number . . . and then maintain; the reality is, always listen to your body. If you ever note that you inexplicably lose strength, you need medical evaluation.

The amounts given for various strengtheners are suggestions only. You may find it best to do less at times, or you may find it better to do more. You be the judge.

WALKING WISDOM: Play with the plus+ers, but always keep within your comfort zone, not your lazy zone.

GET SET. GO!

Great Walk plus+ers can be done walking, standing or lying in bed. They can be done alone or with others. They can be done as warm-ups or warm-downs. They can be done when watching television. Whatever works for you.

Taken together, the plus+ers will help you have....

POWER FEET   KNOCKOUT KNEES   HIP HIPS
A MOBILE TRUNK   HAPPY SHOULDERS

PLUS+ERS TO DO WALKING

-FOR POWER FEET AND KNOCKOUT KNEES

PAUSE WALK *For strengthening your shin muscles and stretching your back leg muscles.*

Before heel contact, pause with your foot about 3 inches off the ground and your toes pointed toward the sky. Count three slowly. As you count, try closing the space between your toes and shin.

Alternate 1 minute of pause walking with 1 minute of regular walking. Repeat three times.

LITTLE PIGGY PULL-UPS

As you walk, concentrate on raising your little toe at heel contact. Alternate 1 minute of Little Piggy Pull-Ups with 1 minute of regular walking. Repeat three times.

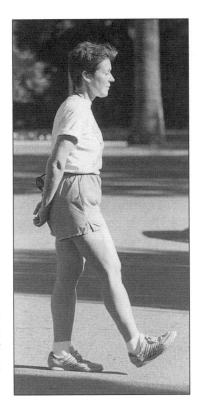

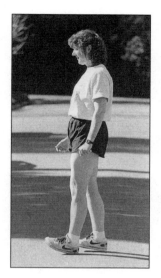

HEEL WALK

Walk on the back edges of your heels. Toes are kept high in the air and legs are straight. Heel walk 15 to 60 seconds.

-FOR HIP HIPS AND A MOBILE TRUNK

DOUBLE CROSS

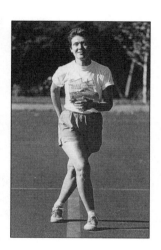

Walk and cross each foot in succession over a real or imaginary line so that the outside of each foot is parallel to the line. Take a large enough step so that your hip goes forward with your crossing leg and foot. Do this plus+er for one minute, rest, and repeat for one minute.

ROCK-A-CRADLE

Make a cradle by laying the palm of your right hand on the back of your left hand. Swing the cradle at your right side so that your elbows go behind and in front of your body. Have your head turned to the right as you walk. Make 15 to 30 full swings. Shift the cradle to the left side. Turning your head towards the left, do 15 to 30 more.

-FOR HAPPY SHOULDERS

ROLLING SHRUGS

Rolling Shrugs and Wings can be done walking as well as standing.

(Think of the backstroke in swimming.) As you walk, roll one shoulder and then the other in backward circles in sync with your steps. Synchronize the bottom point of each shoulder roll with your heel contact. Start with 20, both sides, and increase to 50 or more.

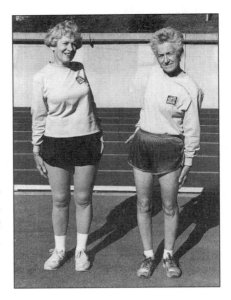

WINGS

With finger tips on the outside points of your shoulders, draw full backward circles with both elbows as you walk. As each elbow brushes your waist, contact the ground with your heel. Start with 20 and increase to 50 or more.

If you are unable to make a full circle with your elbow, do what you can. As you limber up, the size of your circle will increase.

PLUS+ERS TO DO STANDING

-FOR POWER FEET

THUMPER TOES

Keeping your heel on the ground, raise your toes off the ground and lower them to tap the ground. Toe tap quickly for 10 to 15 seconds with each foot. Gradually increase the time duration until you are able to tap for 30 seconds with each foot.

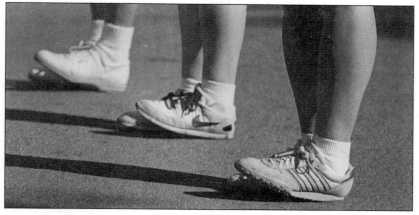

Toe Tapping

DIZZY FEET

Draw circles in the air with your big toes for 10 to 15 seconds with each foot. Gradually increase the time to 30 seconds or longer.

THE SCHOLARLY DIGIT

Draw the alphabet in the air with the big toe of each foot. Make the letters large. Be sure both big digits become equally scholarly.

HELLO, SHINS!

Standing with your arms outstretched at shoulder height, alternate raising the toes of your right foot and left foot as high off the ground as you can. Keep your legs straight. Do these toe raises 10 times with both feet. Rest 15 counts and repeat. Gradually increase to 20 times.

Your shin muscles may let you know they are being worked by a sensation of burning and spasm. If they do, what you feel is their protest at being used after so many years of neglect.

SHINS, AGAIN

With your back resting against a wall and with your heels 10 to 12 inches from the wall, alternate raising and lowering your toes. Keep your legs straight, and let your hips move up and down with your toes. Begin with 10 to 15 seconds and gradually increase to one minute as your tolerance allows.

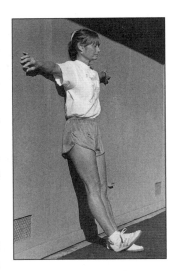

CALF STRETCHES

With the palms of your hands against a support, lean forward with your right leg bent and your left leg extended behind you. Keep both feet flat on the ground. Lean until you feel a pleasant stretching in the calf muscles of your extended leg. Hold this stretch 15 seconds or longer. Do two times each leg.

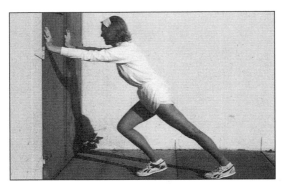

-FOR KNOCKOUT KNEES

ANTI-BEND I *For knee straightening.*

Standing on your right leg, place your left heel on a raised support, toes up. The support should be high enough to allow comfortable stretching from ankle to lower back. To increase the stretch, lean toward your toes, or move the fingers of your left hand down your shin toward your toes. When you feel an easy stretching, hold 15 to 30 seconds. Switch sides. Repeat each leg. (You do not want to feel any sharp pulling in your muscles.)

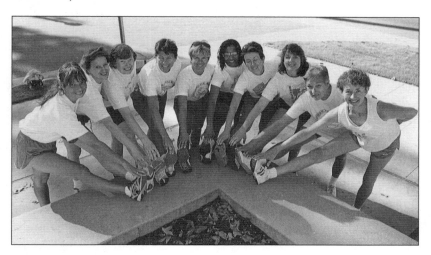

ANTI-BEND II

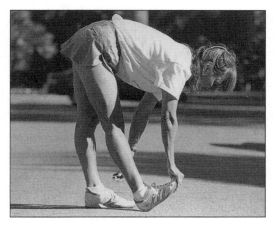

Standing on your left leg, extend your right leg in front of your body and point your toes up in the air. With your supporting knee bent or straight, lean over and touch your toes with your right hand. If you can't reach your toes, reach as far as you can comfortably. Hold for a count of 20. Switch sides. Stretch both legs two times.

KNEEL-SIT *For strengthening the quadriceps.*

Kneeling on the ground, keep your back straight and head up. Now, sit back on your heels and come back up to your knees. Do this 15 times or more.

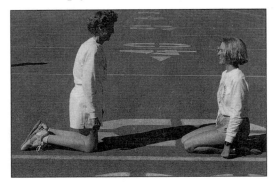

If you have knee problems, this plus+er is not appropriate. Otherwise, it is easy and effective.

LOOK, MA, NO CHAIR! *For strong quads .*

With your back flat against a wall, "sit down" as though a chair was under you. Ideally, your thighs should be parallel to the ground and your lower legs parallel to the wall; however, you can "sit" with less of a knee bend. Start "sitting" for 5 to 15 seconds. Goal-To hold this position for 1 minute.

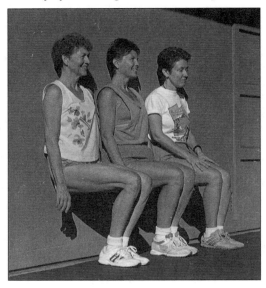

To get back up on your feet, put the palms of your hands flat against the wall behind you and push yourself up.

KNEE PATS *For the quads again.*

With your elbows bent and close to your waist, extend your forearms. The fingers of your hands are outstretched, and your palms are down and parallel to the ground. Marching in place, raise your left knee to touch your left palm and your right knee to touch your right palm. Keep the supporting leg straight. March 20 to 60 seconds.

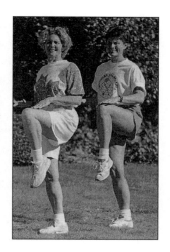

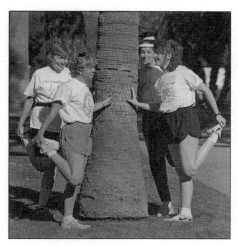

SUPER QUAD STRETCH

Hold on to a support with your right hand. Bending your left leg up behind you, grab your foot with your left hand. Hold for a slow count of 15 or more. Switch sides. Do two times each leg.

VASTUS MEDIALIS STRENGTHENER *For strengthening the vastus medialis muscle, the quadriceps muscle that helps straighten your leg the last 15 degrees.*

TEST: First, let's find your vastus medialis muscle. Extend your right leg on a bed (couch or floor) with a rolled towel under the knee. Put the fingers of your left hand about one inch above and just to the inside of your right knee cap. Push down against the towel with your right knee. You should feel your vastus medialis harden under your finger tips. If you don't, move your fingers around a bit. If you still don't, you definitely need to strengthen this muscle.

STRENGTHENERS *For both legs.*

1 With a rolled towel under your knee, extend one leg on a bed (couch of floor). Push the towel down with your knee 10 to 25 times slowly.

2 Sit in a chair with one heel resting on the floor and leg extended. Push down gently with your knee 10 to 25 times slowly.

3 Sit on a raised surface (table or counter). Extend one leg out in front and flex your foot toward your shin maximally, count 3, relax foot, and repeat to tolerance.

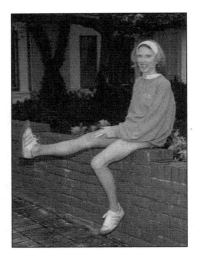

Vastus Medialis

ANTI-KNOCK I *For knock-knees.*

Walk with both feet turned way out for one or two minutes. Increase the amount of time you walk this way gradually as you will be working the inside leg muscles that are weak. They will become sore if you overdo.

ANTI-KNOCK II

Stand with toes pointed forward. Roll your feet to the outside edges and tighten the leg muscles so that you create space between your thighs. Return to start position and repeat. Roll out 15 times, rest for a count of 5 and repeat 15 times. Gradually increase to 50 as tolerance allows.

Variation: Roll to outside, hold for count of 5, release and repeat 10 times. Gradually increase hold to a count of 10.

FOR HIP HIPS AND A MOBILE TRUNK

UPSIDE DOWN SOCIALIZER

With feet apart and knees bent, lean over from the waist letting your head and arms hang down. Maintain a comfortable stretch for a slow count of 20 to 30. As your muscles relax, your head will go lower and increase the stretch naturally.

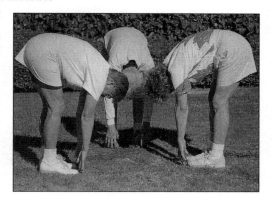

ELVIS THE PELVIS

Standing with feet apart and hands on your hips, rotate your pelvis in a circle 10 times. Reverse directions 10 times.

FINGERS TO TOES

With your back against a wall and heels away from the wall 6 to 12 inches, stretch your arms above your head and then lean over so your fingers hang toward your toes or touch your toes. The objective is to give a

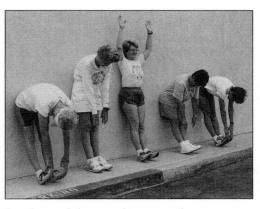

gentle stretch to your back and buttocks muscles, not to touch your toes. Hold for a count of 15 to 30. Rise up and repeat 1 or 2 times.

FIGURE EIGHTS

Holding on to a support, stand on one leg. Draw a figure 8 with the toe of your free foot. Draw the top part of the 8 in front of you and the bottom part of the 8 behind you. Gradually increase the size of the 8 so that your hip rotates fully in the back and front. Do figure 8's ten to twenty times each leg. (Reminder, if you have arthritis in your hip, do this to your own tolerance.)

SITTING CROSSOVERS

Sitting with a back support, cross your right leg over a bent left leg. Place the outside of your right foot against your left thigh and hug the knee to your body. Hold for a slow count of 15 to 30. Switch legs. Do two sets.

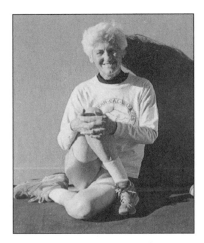

PRAYING SOLES

Sitting with or without a back support, put the soles of your feet together and rest your elbows on the inside of your legs. You will feel a stretch in the groin area. You can regulate this stretch by moving your feet closer to, or farther from, your body. The closer, the more intense the stretch. Count 30 or more, release and repeat.

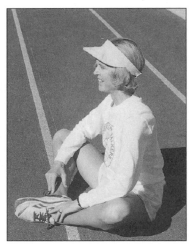

FOR A MOBILE TRUNK

KEGELS *For strengthening the perineal muscles.*

(The perineal muscles are at the lower end of your trunk between your thighs. They support your internal abominal organs.)

Kegels basically involve tightening the perineal muscles by squeezing the openings of the urethra, vagina and rectum just as nature sometimes demands. If you want to feel these muscles working, stop your urine in midstream and hold. As you tighten your perineals, tighten your abdominal muscles as well.

1 Squeeze the openings of your urethra, vagina and rectum. Hold for a count of 3 and release. Do 15 times. Increase to 25 times.

2 Squeeze and release as above, but in rapid succession for a count of 15 to 30. Increase to 50 or more.

Do Kegels four times a week, every day or many times a day. They can be done standing, sitting or lying. Your ability to tighten or squeeze will develop with practice. At first, you may not feel much of anything happening, but you will as the muscles get stronger.

WALL PRESSES *For strengthening the abdominal muscles.*

Stand against a wall with your heels, hips and shoulders touching. Suck in your lower abdominal muscles so your back flattens against the wall. Hold for a count of 5 and release. Repeat 5 times.

Variation: Stand against a wall with your heels, hips and shoulders touching. As you pull in

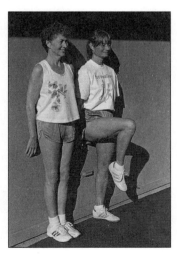

your abdominals, raise your left knee waist high. Hold for a count of 5 and lower your leg. Now raise your right knee waist high, hold for a count of 5 and lower. Do 3 sets.

GENTLE TWIST *For lower back flexibility.*

Standing with arms out shoulder height, gently rotate your body to the right and to the left. Do 10 to 20 times.

LOVABLE KNEES I *Another for the lower back.*

Seated, hug your knees to your chest. Hold as long as you want.

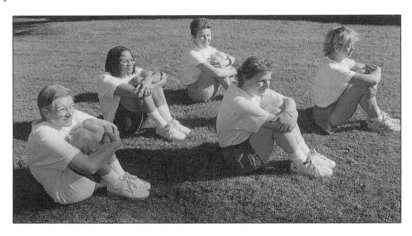

FOR HAPPY SHOULDERS

WINDMILLS *Windmills can be done walking.*

Singles: With your left arm resting across your stomach, rotate your right arm in backward circles 10 times with your palm out. Bring your arm up close to your ear and keep your elbow straight. As your arm goes behind you, let your hip turn back so that you can get a full rotation. (If you keep your hips facing front, your rotating arm will go out rather than back.) Switch and do windmills with other arm.

Doubles: Do double windmills slowly and gently. Make backward circles with both arms alternating their up and down positions. Again, bring your arms up close to your ears with palms out and keep your elbows straight. Remember to let your hips turn back during the backward phase of the arm rotation. Do 5 to 10 doubles at first and increase to tolerance.

BACK SCRATCHER

With one hand reaching over your shoulder and the other reaching up from your waistline, scratch your back with your fingers. It will feel so good you won't have to count 15. Switch arm positions.

HALF HUGS

With your right hand, reach across to your left shoulder and extend your hand as far around to the back of the shoulder as possible. Hold for a count of 15. Do the same with your other arm, extending your left hand behind your right shoulder. Repeat two times.

PLUS+ERS TO DO IN BED

FOR POWER FEET

UNDERCOVER MANEUVERS

Lying on your back in bed, alternate flexing and straightening your ankles under a loosely tucked-in sheet. Don't be surprised if you feel your shin muscles protesting quite quickly. Don't be surprised to hear some other kinds of protest if you have a pillow mate.

Do these undercover flexions 5 times, each foot. Rest and do them 5 more times. Gradually work up to 15 times.

MORE UNDERCOVER MANEUVERS

Lying on your back in bed under a lightly tucked in top sheet for resistance, make 10 circles with one foot, 10 circles with the other, and 10 circles with both feet. Reverse direction and do another set of 10 circles.

FOR A MOBILE TRUNK

ABDOMINAL TUCKS   *For strengthening the abdominal muscles.*

1 When lying in bed on your back, slowly press your low back against your mattress. Hold for a count of 5 and release. Do 5 to 10 times and relax. Increase to 20.

2 Do 10 to 15 low back presses quickly.

During the day, if you develop lower back pain, do back presses against a wall, a chair or the driver's seat in your car. This maneuver can bring surprising relief. (Doing Kegels can also help.)

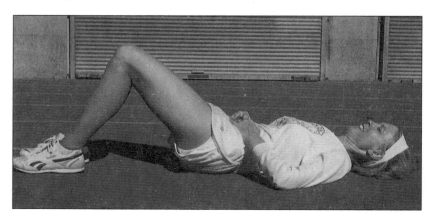

LOVABLE KNEES II   *For stretching back and buttocks muscles.*

Lying on your back, bend your knees and hug them over your chest. Hold 15 to 60 seconds. Relax and repeat. This is a gentle, soothing lower back stretch.

SOW BUG *For strengthening and stretching.*

Lying on your back, bring your knees up to your chest while raising your head up off the mattress to meet them. Hug your knees and bury your face in them. Count 10 to 30. Release and repeat 2 to 3 times.

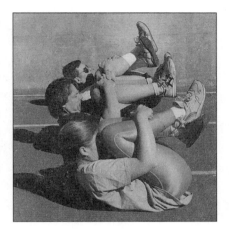

CURLS *For strengthening abdominals.*

Lie on your back with knees bent and slightly apart. Tightening your abdominals, curl your head up off the mattress and extend your arms toward your knees.

At first just do one curl, holding it for a count of 3. Gradually add another curl until you can do 5 curls consecutively, counting to 3. Gradually increase the holding count from 3 to 10. When you can do ten curls for 10 counts each, pat yourself on the back!

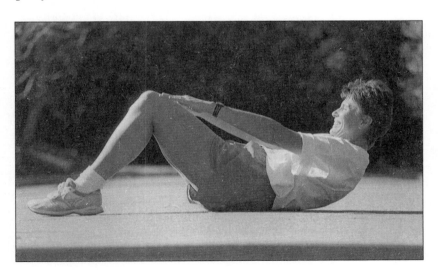

BUN STRETCHER

Lie on your back with your arms flat against your bed. With your left leg straight, bend your right knee and drape it over your left knee until you feel a stretch in your buns and lower back. Count 15 or more and switch legs. Do 2 or 3 times.

GRASSHOPPER LEGS I *For stretching groin muscles.*

Lying on your back, bring the soles of your feet together keeping the sides of your feet on the mattress. Hold for a count of 15 or more. Relax and repeat.

GRASSHOPPER LEGS II

Lying on your back, grasp your feet with your hands and bring the soles of your feet together in the air. Hold for a count of 15 or more, relax and repeat.

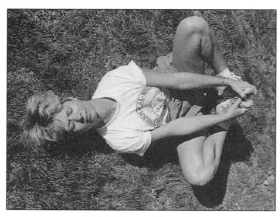

Grasshopper Legs II

FOR HAPPY SHOULDERS AND NECK

STRETCH I

Press your left cheek against your mattress and hold for a count of 15. Repeat with your right cheek. Do 2 or 3 times each cheek. If you have arthritis in your neck, do this stretch carefully.

STRETCH II

Sit on the edge of your bed and look over your right shoulder for a count of 15, and then look over your left shoulder for a count of 15. Repeat.

STRETCH III

Touch your chin to your chest and hold for a count of 10. Now, draw a circle with your chin. Do not bend your head back and compress your cervical spine. Do 5 to 10 times.

WHOLE BODY STRETCH

Lie on your back with arms and legs outstretched. Reach out with your fingers and toes. Hold for a count of 15 or more. Release and repeat 3 times.

When you have done this stretch 3 times, you should feel quite relaxed. Enjoy the feeling.

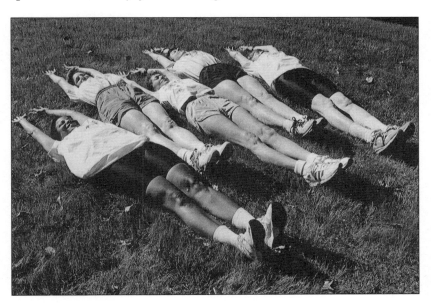

PLUS+ING
And Payoffs

✧

A PEP TALK

Fitness freaks can be hyperbores. They know they know, and they want you to know they know EVERYTHING. So let's come to an understanding. It's okay to avoid fitness freaks. (Their mothers love them.)

However, if you ever feel that you don't care about your own fitness, you may be suffering the triple E crisis. Perhaps you have slipped into one of life's holes and feel that you lack the Energy to make the Effort to crawl out. And, of course, you have zillions of Excuses.

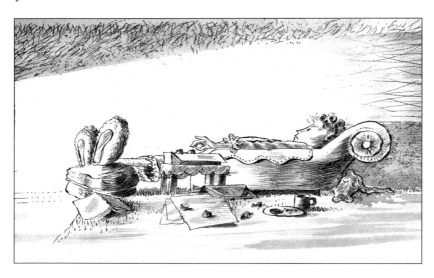

WALKING DYNAMICS TEST 101-A

A SAMPLER OF EXCUSES

I would like to plus my walk, but...

> I don't have time.
> I'm too busy.
> I'm too tired.
> I'm lazy.

I don't feel well.
I'm stressed out.
I'm depressed.
It's too cold.
It's too hot.
I hate exercise.
I have a sick relative.

If every so often you nod "Amen" to one or more of the above, that's okay. Excuses are 100% human, and you qualify! But remind yourself quickly that you will be a big loser if you leave your walk unplused. You risk losing valuable opportunities for fulfilling your cherished wishes.

THE ENERGY-EFFORT FACTOR

Energy is in the bubbles of champagne. It is in the plume of steam from a geyser. It is in the flow of electricity lighting the dark and in the nurturing warmth of the sun. Energy is the elixir of the fountain of youth — the element that gives a woman's maturity excitement and makes a good walk Grrrreat.

Becoming a Great Walker starts with a small investment of energy — the little mental kick that gets you started plus+ing your walk. Making this investment regularly may require more will power some days than others. It may require a little mulish stick-to-itiveness, but the dividends from practicing the plus+ing tips soon start pouring in.

As you become familiar with the technique, you will notice that your walk feels a little easier and a little smoother than it did before. You will notice more strength and control over your body. And the payoffs will start multiplying as you replace old walking habits with new ones. There can be moments when you feel as though you have tapped into a bonanza that is spilling over into every aspect of your life.

Let's see how this multiplication of rewards can happen as we review the tips and payoffs of the plus+ing process.

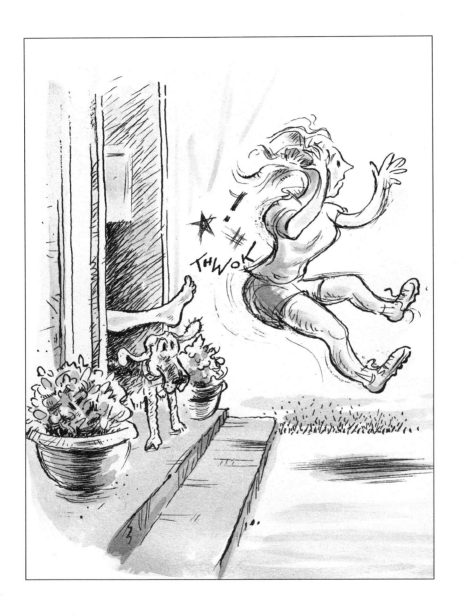

FORWARD POSTURE AND GRAVITY

PLUS+ING

+ Shift your weight to the front of your feet.
  You will have a slight forward lean from your ankles.
+ Hold your head up.
+ Keep your chest lifted.
+ Keep your shoulders relaxed.
+ Tuck in your abdomen and buttocks.

PAYOFFS

$ Makes walking easier.
$ Aids faster walking.
$ Helps communicate self-confidence and purpose.
$ Supports being friendly.
$ Assists self-assertion.

FOOTWORK

PLUS+ING

+ Raise your toes just before heel contact.
+ Contact the ground with your heel close to your body.
+ Point your toes forward.
+ Roll along the fleshy bridge of your sole from heel to toe.
+ Push the ground back with the front of your feet and with your toes.

PAYOFFS

$ Strengthens your feet, ankles, and knees.
$ Improves lower extremity circulation.
$ Shapes and slims your calves and thighs.
$ Puts safety in fast walking.
$ Gives your stride rhythm and grace.
$ Adds energy and vitality to your appearance.

STRAIGHT KNEE

PLUS+ING

+ Straighten your knee as you raise your toes.
+ Roll from heel contact to the support position keeping your knee straight (or as straight as possible).

PAYOFFS

$ Gives your leg an attractive line.
$ Empowers your walk by making the leg a firm lever for the rolling, pushing action of the foot.
$ Increases stability and endurance for distance walking.
$ Gives style and poise to your walking appearance.

HIP ROTATION

PLUS+ING

+ Walk from your waist and allow your hips to rotate with the forward and backward movement of your legs.
+ Keep your shoulders relaxed and facing front.
+ Feel an easy twisting in your waist.

PAYOFFS

$ Integrates the movements of your upper body and lower body.
$ Increases your stride length.
$ Eliminates the physical stress of overstriding.
$ Slims your waistline and hips.
$ Energizes your body.
$ Gives a fluid suppleness to your appearance.

THE ARM SWING

PLUS+ING

+ Swing your arms at your sides in the same forward–backward direction as your hips and legs.
+ Bend your elbows, and swing your arms near your waistline to walk fast.
+ Make a full arm swing front and back.
+ Keep your shoulders level and relaxed.

PAYOFFS

$ Provides coordination and balance.
$ Massages tight shoulder muscles.
$ Reduces neck and shoulder pain.
$ Brings a feeling of freedom to your upper body.
$ Gives a pleasing finish to your walking appearance.

THE HEAD

PLUS+ING

+ Keep your head up.
+ Keep your eyes forward.

PAYOFFS

$ Improves balance and coordination.
$ Reduces stress in neck, shoulder and back muscles.
$ Supports a self-confident, "I can" attitude.
$ Facilitates expressing goodwill to others.

YOU CAN HAVE IT ALL

You now have many tips and pointers to add to your roundabout and fitness walking. By plus+ing your posture, feet, knees, hips and arms, you make walking a total body exercise that requires no special equipment except good shoes. You also make walking a truly safe exercise by eliminating those body movements which can lead to chronic aches and pains. And do not overlook rehabilitation and injury prevention. Plus+ing your walk increases the strength and flexibility in your muscles and joints far more than ordinary walking.

By plus+ing your walking appearance, you gain the ability to impress others favorably when it matters most to you. You can present yourself as a person of purpose and poise. You can use your walk to communicate confidence in your worth and ability. On a day-to-day basis, you gain a small, but highly visible skill to aid your career success.

As to your social and romantic life, the bottom line is that plus+ing your walk increases your sex appeal. It gives you ways of energizing your walk to become an eye stopper. If you are single, you can make sure that "he" is aware of you approaching or passing by. If you are married, you can enjoy knowing that your walk nurtures the flames of romance.

The plus+ing process is especially fun for those over fifty. Stereotypes of growing old haunt us all. By plus+ing your walk and doing the stretches and strengtheners, you can avoid the telltale signs of aging. With attention to a healthy diet and proper rest, you can walk as young, or nearly as young, as you feel inside.

Whenever you are plus+ing your walk, focus on the payoffs. Be sure that you never turn practice into work. Would you stop climbing a mountain if you knew there was a large pot of gold at the top waiting for you? You might pause now and then, but it's a good bet that you would be thinking about what to do with the gold, not of the work in reaching it!

You can plus your walk any time. You need no special place. You can practice around the house, going to a neighbor's for coffee and walking your dog. You can practice at your office, store or other place of work as well as going to and from your car. Best of all, you can add the plus+ing technique to your recreational and fitness walks.

Months may pass before you can exchange your old walking habits for new ones, but no one has a stop watch on you. Be patient. Make friends with your body. Enjoy playing with its movements. Gradually you will feel your body shift into the captivating cadence of your own Grrreat Walk!

Remember, there is no one else like you on this planet earth. You are unique and deserve to walk your best. With horns blowing, cymbals crashing and drums rolling, step up and take your place among the world's Great Walkers. YOU can have it ALL!

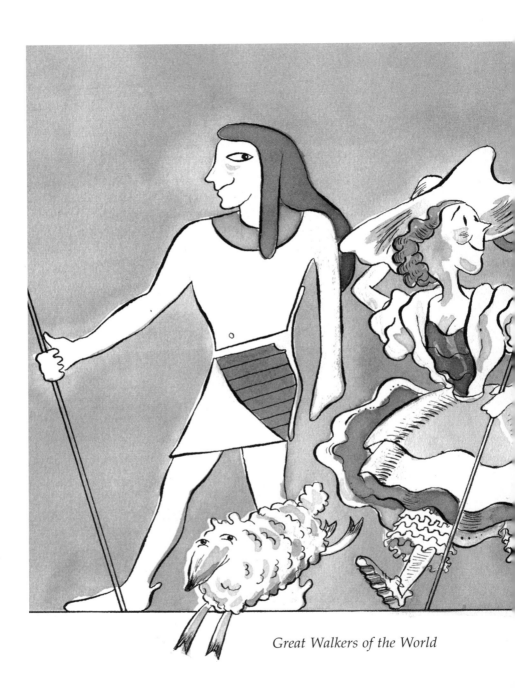

Great Walkers of the World

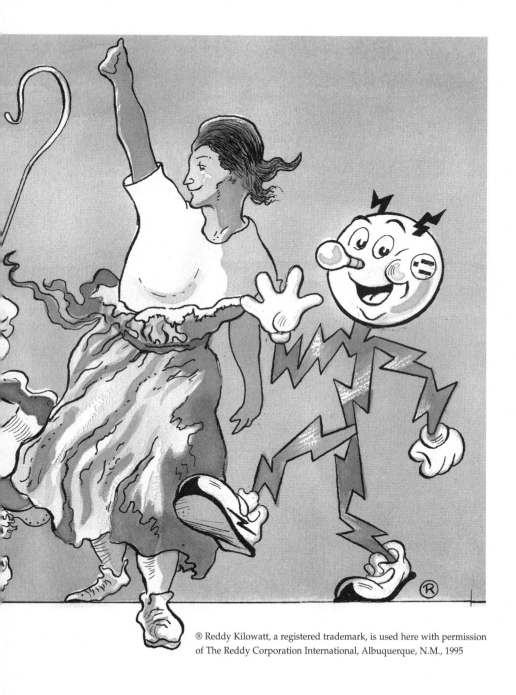

® Reddy Kilowatt, a registered trademark, is used here with permission
of The Reddy Corporation International, Albuquerque, N.M., 1995

Postscript

❧

—— P. S. ——

Knowing that I am a missionary about walking, you will not find it surprising when I say I want to know how you are doing plus+ing your walk. After you've had some success, I hope you will contact me to let me know. I have had my share of frustrations overcoming my own natural problems walking the last few years. I know that it is not easy changing lifelong habits. For that reason, as you succeed, I want to know. I would like the opportunity to congratulate you, as you have much to be congratulated for.

Write me soon. I would like to hear about the challenges you are having as well as the progress you are making.

Sincerely,

Elaine Ward

Walk Plus+ers
1000 San Pasqual, #35
Pasadena, CA 91106-3393
Fax: 818-577-2264

INFORMATION REQUEST

Can we be of any further help to you?
We can send you information about ...

Membership in the Association of
  Walk-Wise Walkers (WWW) _____

Walk Plus+ing Instructional Video _____

Plus+ing Practice Audio Tapes _____

Camp, Clinics, Seminars, Lectures _____

Personal Counselling _____

Corporate Programs & Promotional Setup _____

Additional *Walking Wisdom for Women*
  @ 12.95; shipping 1–3 = $3.00;
  30 cents each additional book.
  Californians add tax $1.07 each _____

Name: _____

Address: _____

City/State/Zip: _____

Wk Phone: _____ Hm Phone: _____

VISA/Mastercard No. _____

Expiration Date _____

Walk Plus+ers, 1000 San Pasqual, #35, Pasadena, CA 91106-3393,
Tel/Fax: 818-577-2264. Credit Card orders 1-800-898-5117.
E-Mail: NARWF@aol.com